THE PARENTS' GUIDE
—— TO ——
PERTHES

Understanding Legg-Calvé-Perthes Disease

CHARLES T. PRICE, MD
BETSY MILLER

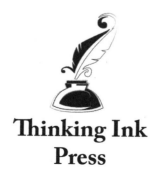

**Thinking Ink
Press**

Published by Thinking Ink Press
P.O. Box 1411, Campbell, California 95009-1411
www.thinkinginkpress.com

First printing, 2015

ISBN 978-1-942480-00-6

Printed in the United States of America.

Library of Congress Control Number: 2014960281

Project Credits

Cover design: Anthony Francis, Loney Grabscheid, Betsy Miller, and Nathan Vargas

Editor: Liza Olmsted

Illustrations: Denise Sutherland

Indexer: Candace Hyatt

Marketing and publicity: Gwen Leong

Contents

Acknowledgments

A number of people stepped up to help with the development of this book. Denise Sutherland, your patience and exactness in creating medically accurate illustrations is greatly appreciated. Thank you Susan Pappas for your help in getting permission to use previously published illustrations and for managing the x-ray images used in this book.

A big thank you to the people who shared their personal stories about Perthes: Donna Colburn Brown, Claudia Giffuni (and Nico), Kate Guscette, Lisa Guscette, Michelle Vance, and Kathy Churchill (and Connor). Catalin Zaharia, we appreciate your insightful comments in response to the early draft of this manuscript.

Liza Olmsted, your careful editing and understanding of the arcane rules involved in citations is greatly appreciated. Casy Hsu, thank you for your fresh perspective on this topic. Gwen Leong, you did a great job helping me spread the word about this book. And an extra special thanks goes out to all the people who participated in the preordering event and to those who contributed extra to make it possible to donate books as resources.

1

Understanding Perthes

Perthes disease, also called Legg-Calvé-Perthes disease, is a condition in which the bone in the ball in a child's hip joint loses its
circulation and becomes brittle. Over time, this causes the bone
to die, but as circulation returns to the joint, new bone gradually
grows in place of the brittle bone. For some children, this process
affects the shape of the ball at the top of the thigh bone, which is
called the femoral head. This can occur in one hip or both hips.

This stoppage of circulation in the hip can occur at any age,
but the problem has different names for other age groups. A
name that applies to any age group is avascular necrosis (AVN).
Avascular means the loss of vascularity (blood flow) and necrosis
means death. So, the term AVN means death of the bone because
of loss of blood supply. However, doctors use a lot of different
terms for this condition. You don't need to remember all of the
names that are used for Perthes. They are explained here and are
also in the glossary for reference. Perthes disease is the most
common name, but you may hear Legg-Calvé-Perthes disease, or
simply AVN because AVN is the medical term for what happened. In fact, AVN can occur in babies and in adults, but it's
only called Perthes in the age group between 2 and 14 years. To
make matters more confusing, AVN in babies and adults is also
called osteonecrosis, or dead bone, in addition to being called
AVN. So, you can see that doctors use many terms to identify
one problem. This is similar to the way we identify ourselves by

our names, full names, nicknames, family relationships, or other terms.

One possible reason that the term Perthes is used for the age group between 4 and 13 is how Perthes affects the shape of the ball at the top of the thigh bone. Babies with AVN always recover with a round ball, but adults never do without treatment. The age between 4 and 13 is unpredictable. Some children in this age group recover without any intervention and others need treatment. So, the first question to ask is: who needs treatment and who doesn't in the age group between 4 and 13 years? Doctors rely on observations, tests, and experience to help decide who needs to be treated and who can be allowed to heal without intervention. We hope that this book will give you some insight into the keys for those decisions.

Hip Anatomy and Blood Supply

A hip joint is a ball-and-socket joint. The top of the thighbone (femur) is round, like a ball, and is called the femoral head. It fits deep inside the hip socket, which is called the acetabulum.

Cartilage covers the surfaces of the joint, and allows it to glide smoothly. Oily fluid inside the joint keeps it lubricated. That fluid is made by the lining of the joint called the synovium. A rim of soft tissue called the labrum surrounds the hip socket: it adds extra support and provides a seal that helps keep the ball inside the socket. Because it is not made of bone, the labrum cannot be seen on x-rays.

In Figure 1, notice that the blood vessels do not cross the growth plate because it is cartilage in the child. This limits the blood supply to the ball until the growth plate turns to bone as an adult. Sometimes Perthes causes the growth plate to turn to bone prematurely and this can cause a growth disturbance.

The blood supply to the hip in children is different from adults. Loss of blood supply leads to Avascular Necrosis (AVN) but that's the term that doctors use to say that the hip is crumbling because it has lost the blood supply—as opposed to damage from trauma, infection, or other conditions. Some special aspects of the anatomy in children between the ages of five and ten years make circulation in the hip joint more precarious. When a child has Perthes, the small blood vessels that give blood to the ball become clotted and that stops the circulation. The ball of the hip does not have overlapping circulation as most other areas of the body, so the hip is especially at risk. Also, the blood vessels of the child's hip need to go around the growth plate and that makes children different from adults where the blood vessels freely travel up the middle of the bone.

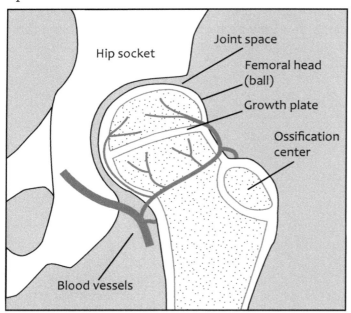

Hip socket

Joint space

Femoral head (ball)

Growth plate

Ossification center

Blood vessels

Figure 1. Normal hip anatomy for a child.

Range of Motion

The hip joint is a ball-and-socket joint like the shoulder, so it can move in all directions. When you walk, the hip joints flex forward and extend backward as you move your legs.[1] The knee also

---

[1] In this book, the word *leg* means the part of the body from the pelvis to the ankle. Doctors may use the term *lower limb* to mean this part of the body, and use the word leg to mean only the part below the knee.

flexes and extends, but it is a hinge joint and can't rotate in all directions.

So why does the hip need to be a ball-and-socket joint? One reason is to allow the leg to swing out to the side (abduction), or inward toward the body (adduction). Actions like riding a horse or squatting involve abduction and adduction. The hip also rotates as you twist at the waist while walking, creating a longer stride. In track and field events, hurdlers twist their hips even more to get one leg stretched out over the hurdle while the other pushes from behind. Ball-and-socket motion is important for understanding Perthes because any limit of rotation or ability to move the hip away from the body causes a limp even though the hip might flex and extend perfectly.

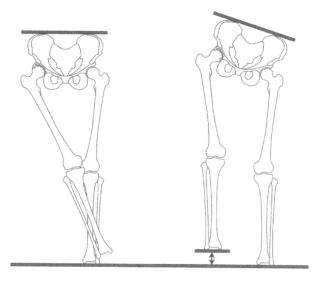

Figure 2. Crossing the legs with a painful limp.

If the ball in the hip joint becomes flat, the flattened ball limits the stride length, and causes the hip to jam when the pelvis tries to rotate.[2] The flattened ball also limits the ability of the leg to swing out to the side. The adductor muscles on the inside of

---

[2] Figure 2 reproduced with permission from D. Paley. Dror Paley, *Principles of Deformity Correction* (New York: Springer, 2002), 737.

the thigh may also be in spasm and prevent the leg from swinging to the normal position while walking or standing.

When the hip is painful, the leg may become stuck when crossing the midline because of muscle spasms or flatness of the ball. Then the child must hike the pelvis to walk and this makes the leg seem shorter than it really is.

Risk Factors and Possible Causes

Perthes is an uncommon disorder that affects more boys than girls in a ratio of five boys for every girl. While girls are less likely to get Perthes, they often have worse cases, or more long-term consequences. One reason is that girls stop growing before boys do, so there isn't as much time for the hip to recover completely. We don't know all the reasons for these differences between boys and girls although the increased activity level of boys has been considered as a possible cause. Perthes is also more common in low-birth weight children and in children with delayed maturity. This means that children with Perthes are often smaller than other children their age. Some children are exceptions to these trends, and that makes it difficult for doctors to be certain about what increases the risk of Perthes. Although several other possible causes of Perthes have been considered, there has been no conclusive evidence that Perthes is caused by parental cigarette smoking, increased blood coagulation, nutritional deficiencies, Attention Deficit Hyperactivity Disorder (ADHD), or kidney abnormalities. Researchers continue to look for causes.

The frequency of Perthes is difficult to estimate because ethnicity and the region in which a child lives seems to affect how common Perthes is even within the same country. About one in 10,000 white children in the USA will get Perthes, but the frequency in Black children is about 1 in 200,000. Asians have a rate of about 1 per 25,000, and Hispanics approximately 1 in 50,000.

Perthes affects children between the ages of 2 and 14 years old, and the peak age at onset is 5 to 7 years. Even the age at onset varies in some regions, and the peak age is older in India than in Europe or the USA. It's not known whether the number of cases of Perthes is increasing or decreasing, but there is evidence in England that the total number of cases is decreasing, perhaps because of improved standards of living over the past fifty years.

Diagnosing Perthes

A diagnosis of Perthes has two parts. The first part is to make sure that the cause of the limp or pain is Perthes and not something else like an infection or an injury. The x-ray findings of Perthes are distinct, so a knowledgeable doctor can usually make the diagnosis based on x-rays. The second part is diagnosing the extent and stage. The extent means the amount of involvement or how much of the ball at the top of the thigh bone is affected. Younger children can tolerate more involvement than older children. Perthes goes through a series of stages. Chapter 2 describes each stage of Perthes and also discusses how the amount of involvement affects treatment.

The extent is hard to determine early in the course of Perthes when treatment decisions need to be made. Taking x-rays periodically helps because the extent becomes clearer as the bone changes. However, observing and waiting too long to intervene may decrease the chances of a good outcome. This is a major dilemma of Perthes: early treatment gives the best results, but it's not always easy to know who needs treatment in early stages.

To find out the stage, doctors use the child's history, physical exams, and x-rays. The history tells the doctor how long the child has been in pain or limping. Limping is a way to avoid pain, so doctors consider limping to be a sign of pain avoidance. Pain or limping for less than six months usually means the disease is still in the early stages.

X-Rays

In the early stages of Perthes, the x-rays may show few changes except for a crack under the joint surface, some increased whiteness of the bone, or a slight change in the shape of the ball. Doctors use x-rays to monitor Perthes as it progresses. After a few months, the ball in the hip joint shows a moth-eaten appearance on x-rays as the dead bone is absorbed so that new bone can grow. In the later stages of Perthes, the ball is soft and may start to fragment or flatten and slip out of the joint sideways. The length of time the child has had pain or a limp plus the changes on the x-rays help determine the stage of Perthes.

It might seem that nuclear bone scans, CT scans, or standard MRI scans could reveal the extent of Perthes, but these methods tend to overestimate how much of the joint is affected. Plain x-rays are still the best method for estimating the extent of involvement of the ball, but this is an area of active research.

Concerns About X-Ray Hazards

X-rays are the rays that generate the image similar to the way that light rays generate an image in a digital camera or on photographic paper. Pictures of friends and family are called photographs. The images produced by x-rays are properly called radiographs, but we call these images x-rays even though the x-rays are the beams of energy that caused the images to appear.

In years gone by, lots of x-ray energy was required to produce the images on plastic films. Today's images are produced digitally with computer enhancement so the amount of x-rays needed to produce a good radiograph is very small. The same changes have occurred in photography, where today's digital cameras—especially video cameras—can take good pictures indoors without much light. Similar technology enhances the x-ray images.

The amount of x-ray exposure with digital imaging is so low that it is usually best to avoid shielding of the genital organs so that the best x-rays can be obtained on the first set of x-rays (radiographs). This is safe and standard in most offices or hospitals where children are treated. If you are in doubt, it doesn't hurt to ask the doctor if his x-ray equipment is digital or if he is using "rare earth" x-ray exposures. Either of those has very low irradiation. CT scans have a lot of x-ray exposure but MRI has none.

In the past, shielding was recommended because ovaries and testes are sensitive to radiation. A recent study[3] of pelvic x-rays of children found that the shields were placed incorrectly most of the time, and that the radiation exposure with modern x-ray equipment is very small. The study concluded that it might be better to stop the shielding.

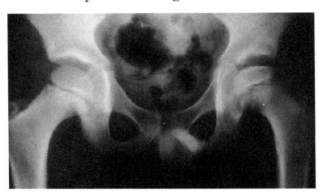

Figure 3. Early Perthes. The hip on your right has Perthes.

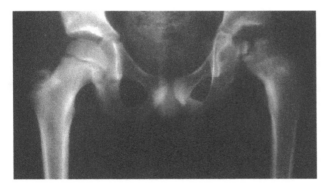

Figure 4. Later Perthes in the same child as Figure 3.

Interpreting X-Rays

X-rays taken in the early course of Perthes may only show that one hip is whiter and a little flatter than the normal hip. Initially,

[3] Marij J. Frantzen et al., "Gonad Shielding in Paediatric Pelvic Radiography: Disadvantages Prevail Over Benefit", Insights into Imaging 3.1 (2012): 23, http://www.ncbi.nlm.nih.gov/pmc/articles/PMC3292647/.

it is hard to detect this difference but the whiteness becomes more pronounced after a few weeks. The whiteness is because the blood stops circulating, and fluids that are rich in calcium seep into the spongy bone. Limping also leads to bone loss around the dead bone and this makes the contrast more apparent. The area of white bone is the first clue to the extent of Perthes. When this is clearly seen, it usually shows how much of the ball is affected. A small central area of whiteness is less worrisome than complete involvement of the ball where the whole ball is white. (The anatomy of a child's hip is shown in "Figure 1. Normal hip anatomy for a child." on page 3.)

Sometimes a crack below the surface of the joint is visible where the brittle dead bone has broken. This break usually causes some pain for the child and may be the first sign of Perthes. The length and location of the crack has been used to classify the severity of Perthes with the Salter-Thompson method. (See "Perthes Classifications" on page 37.)

Unfortunately, it's not a reliable method because the x-rays rarely show the whole crack, and may not show the crack at all. Imagine shining a light through a crack in a wall. If the light isn't lined up perfectly with the crack, then the light won't shine through to the other side. If the x-ray beams don't line up with the crack in the ball then the x-ray beam won't shine through onto the radiograph.

Interpreting x-rays of Perthes is more about what you don't see than what you do see, because the changes visible on x-ray lag behind the process by four to six months. As time goes by, the white bone is taken away by blood vessels that grow into the ball to help it recover. Then the ball begins to look moth-eaten because the blood vessels don't show up on the x-rays. The areas of bone that look like they are gone have been replaced by blood vessels and cartilage as part of the healing process. The ball becomes soft and likely to collapse where the white bone is disappearing during this stage. If only a small part of the ball is affected, then the normal areas will give support and keep the ball from collapsing.

Another area that doesn't show up on the x-ray is the joint space. This is the area between the ball and the socket, but it's not actually a space because it is filled with cartilage on the surface of the ball and the lining of the socket. The bone has blood, but the cartilage surface does not. When the bone loses blood supply, the bone becomes brittle and no longer supports the cartilage surface.

If the ball collapses, it becomes very white and thin and the ball does not take up as much space in the socket. This allows the ball to move upward and slide out of the socket sideways. Some x-ray measurements can help determine if this is happening. Perhaps the best way is to look at something called Shenton's line.

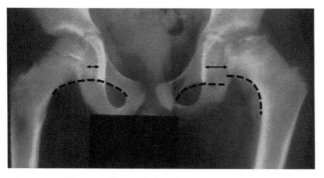

Figure 5. Shenton's line is broken.

Shenton's line is the smooth arc across the bottom of the hip joint where the ball is in the socket. Figure 5 shows a broken Shenton's line on the side with Perthes.

Arthrogram (X-Ray with Dye)

Arthrography, also called an arthrogram, is an x-ray taken after dye is injected into a joint to show more detail than can be seen in a plain x-ray. Anesthesia is used during this procedure. The hip is always round at the beginning of Perthes, so arthrography has little role during the early stages. An arthrogram is generally used if the hip has begun to slide out of the socket sideways to see if the hip can be put back into the socket.

The arthrogram also helps show whether the ball is too flat to recover with standard surgery or by putting the child in a cast for an extended period of time. An MRI may show the flatness of the femoral head, but general anesthesia during arthroscopy relaxes the muscle spasms and lets the doctor determine if the hip is too far out of the socket to go back in. If the hip cannot be put back into the socket, then salvage procedures may be needed.

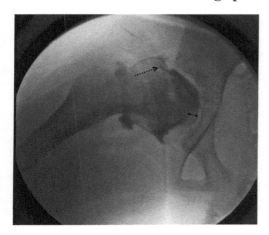

Figure 6. Hip arthrogram.

In Figure 6, the dye in the joint is black and the dotted arrow points to a dent in the ball that is hooked on the edge of the socket. The dye shows up between the ball and the edge of the socket because the ball cannot be put back into the socket completely. When Perthes has reached this stage, doctors call it "hinge abduction" and containment is rarely possible or successful. (See "Hinge Abduction" on page 20.)

Computed Tomography (CT)

Computed tomography (CT) is commonly called a CAT scan. This is rarely needed for children with Perthes, and it exposes the child to many more x-rays than other types of imaging. Newer CT machines have less radiation, but it's worthwhile to question your doctor about alternatives whenever a CT is recommended.

Current CT technology does not accurately show how much of the ball is affected by Perthes. During a CT, the x-ray beam moves around the body so that images can be seen from many angles. The final images show "slices" of the area being scanned.

Magnetic Resonance Imaging (MRI)

In Perthes, the standard MRI may be helpful to diagnose Perthes. MRI does not use x-rays. It uses a strong magnetic field and radio waves to create images of tissues. This allows the doctor see the ligaments, muscles, and tendons (also called soft tissue) around a joint much more clearly than on an x-ray. An MRI lets the doctor see the joint surface and the joint shape. It's necessary to stay very still for 15–20 minutes while the MRI is being done, so babies and children usually need sedation or general anesthesia for an MRI so that they stay still and the images are clear.

Standard MRI is not very helpful to guide treatment. This is because the standard MRI tends to overestimate or underestimate the extent of the damage. However, perfusion MRI, also called contrast MRI, is more sensitive in detecting how much of the femoral head has lost its blood flow. In perfusion MRI, a contrast solution is given through a vein before obtaining the MRI. Since the contrast goes to the area of the femoral head that has blood flow, it shows the area without blood flow as a dark region.

One shortcoming of MRI is that the hip cannot be moved around like it can during an arthrogram (x-ray with dye), so an arthrogram is usually preferred in later stages of Perthes to determine whether the ball can be contained in the socket. However, in some situations the MRI can help define the shape of the ball if the child can hold still without general anesthesia.

The doctor might recommend an MRI with dye injected into the hip joint. This is called an MR arthrogram and is very rarely used for Perthes. An MR arthrogram may be needed later if a child has pain after the Perthes has run its course and the hip is not round. In these cases the soft tissues around the joint may be damaged and imaging may need dye in the joint to enhance the MRI. For instance, a teen who is thought to have a tear in the labrum (the soft rim of cartilage that surrounds the hip joint) might need an MR arthrogram. Sometimes a high-resolution MRI machine can reveal more detail about the joint and avoid the dye injection, but not all facilities have the highest resolution machines. If dye is used, a local anesthetic is injected into the hip joint first, then the contrast material is injected.

2

Considerations for the Treatment Plan

Three main variables influence the treatment of Perthes:

- The stage, or progression. In other words, how long the Perthes has been going on.

- The extent. This is the amount of the ball at the top of the thigh bone that is involved or abnormal.

- The age of the child at the onset of Perthes, when pain or limping began. This is the most important variable that determines the outcome of Perthes.

Young children have very thick cartilage on the surface of the ball, so the joint space looks thicker on the x-ray. Young children benefit from this extra thickness because it helps prevent collapse even when the bone underneath is dead and being replaced. This thick cartilage is like thick walls of a tire that can help keep the tire from collapsing even when the air goes out of it. By age eight, the cartilage surface of the ball is thinner, so collapse is more likely even when the area of dead bone is smaller.

This difference in cartilage thickness may be one reason why younger children have better outcomes without treatment. Also, when collapse does occur in younger children, they have more years of growth remaining for the hip to remodel and return to a rounder shape. In this context, remodel means that the bones grow into a more normal shape and alignment. The time remaining for growth is less in girls than in boys, so girls should be treated as if they were a little older than a boy the same age.

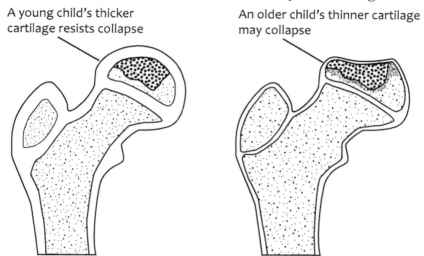

A young child's thicker cartilage resists collapse

An older child's thinner cartilage may collapse

Figure 7. Perthes cartilage thickness by age.

Stage or Progression

All diseases go through stages, and Perthes is no different. The onset stage is when the child first begins to limp or complain of pain. That is followed by a series of other stages as the body attempts to remove the damaged bone and grow new bone.

These stages occur because the dead bone is strong but it tends to weaken over time as small cracks accumulate in the bone. Because the bone is dead, it cannot mend these cracks. This is the reason why a fracture develops in the early stage of Perthes. When the blood flow begins to grow back, the femoral head is further weakened by cells that remove the dead bone.

Muscle forces during a child's activities or exercise cause pressures on the hip joint that are 2.5 to 4 times greater than body weight. This is one of the reasons why some doctors advocate crutch walking early in the disease to lessen the impact of walking on the femoral head.

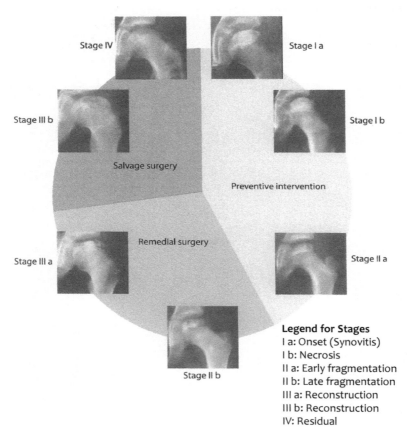

Figure 8. Perthes stages in a child who recovered without treatment. Diagram courtesy of Orthopedic Clinics of North America.

Onset Stage (Synovitis Stage)

The earliest stage is called the onset stage or the synovitis stage. The child begins to have pain and limp. Sometimes the child doesn't complain of pain because the limp relieves weight on the hip. In this case, the limp is one way the body is trying to minimize the harm. The damage in this stage is caused when the small blood vessels to the center of the hip stop working.

Even though the hip bone has lost its blood supply, the bone stays strong for many weeks. During this period the child may experience some pain or limp, but the pain is usually mild and x-rays appear normal. The synovitis stage may last a few weeks or months, but rarely more than three months.

Necrosis Stage

After a few weeks, the bone becomes brittle and small cracks occur. These cracks can be seen on x-rays because the affected bone becomes whiter due to microscopic fractures. The necrosis stage is the first stage that is visible on x-ray. Sometimes a crescent sign (a crescent-shaped crack) and a break can be seen just under the joint surface. This break is often painful enough to warrant a trip to the doctor.

This stage may last four to six months as the damaged bone becomes more visible. The portion of the bone that lost its blood supply is dead. The dead bone stays in the joint and stays brittle until the next stage starts.

Fragmentation Stage

The fragmentation stage represents the body's attempt to repair itself. The brittle bone that lost its blood supply needs to be removed so the body can grow new, living bone in its place. Microscopic blood vessels grow into the dead bone. The dead bone begins to dissolve so that new bone can grow. On x-rays, the ball looks like Swiss cheese with patchy holes, or has a moth-eaten appearance. It may be alarming to parents to watch the bone disappear, but this process is necessary for the bone to repair itself.

The biggest problem during the fragmentation stage is that the bone is at the greatest risk of collapse, and that can permanently deform the ball. This risk of collapse is the basis of the major principle of early treatment: *containment*. This means that the ball is contained in the hip socket so that the socket can act as a mold to keep the ball round while the dead bone is absorbed and new bone grows.

Many methods of containment are used, but all have the same goal of keeping the ball in the socket during the fragmentation stage. The earlier containment begins, the better the outcome. This is because if the ball flattens and collapses, that creates more space between the ball and the socket. The ball can shift and move outside of the hip socket. Then the edge of the hip socket mashes on the flattened ball and flattens it even more. It's best to keep the ball inside the socket before it starts to collapse and shift. The fragmentation stage may last from six months to one year as all the white, dead bone is absorbed. Containment only works as a treatment when it begins before the ball collapses, but the ball does not collapse in every case of Perthes. For these reasons, deciding which child with Perthes should be treated and which one can be watched remains a decision-making dilemma for doctors. (See "Containment Methods" on page 39.)

Reconstitution Stage

The reconstitution stage occurs when all the white, dead bone has dissolved. At this stage, the shape of the ball is permanent. Containment cannot restore it to a round shape. On x-rays, the ball may still appear to have holes in it, but those holes are filled with hard cartilage that will become bone. This cartilage is very strong and will not lose its shape, but it looks clear on x-rays as if the ball has small holes in it. On x-rays, the visible bone in and around those holes is the same gray color as the normal bone of the pelvis instead of looking like the white specks of dead bone seen previously.

It's sometimes difficult for doctors to tell when the reconstitution stage has begun because the ball still looks like Swiss cheese on x-rays. The way to tell is by the length of time the child has had Perthes and also by some of the other x-ray findings. The reconstitution stage is almost always present by 18 months after the first onset of pain or limp. Also, by this time, the ball on the affected hip is usually larger than the other hip. Doctors can generally recognize the reconstitution stage by comparing old x-rays to see if all the dead, white bone is gone, by seeing if the ball has enlarged, and by estimating how long the process has been going on. Recognizing this stage is important because after the reconstitution stage has begun, containment is no longer an effective treatment.

The reconstitution stage may take two or three years for all the cartilage to turn to bone, but the child can resume full activities during this time when the round, slightly enlarged shape of the ball is becoming visible on x-rays. The cartilage and bone are living and healthy with enough strength to support activities. If the ball has grown back in a flattened shape or displaced position, the child's activities might need to be restricted.

Residual Stage

The final stage is the residual stage. This occurs when all the cartilage has been replaced by bone and the entire bone surface of the ball has been restored. This is when the final outcome can be judged and measured to predict the long-term risk of arthritis. If the ball is round and the shape of the upper thigh bone is normal, then the long-term outcome is good and no arthritis is expected before the age of 60 years. When the ball is round, but the femoral neck (the part of the thigh bone that connects to the ball) is short, there may be a slight difference in leg length, or a limp, and a risk of arthritis around the age of 50 years. If the limp is bad, then surgery can restore the length of the neck but the round ball will protect the joint from arthritis for many, many years.

Sometimes the ball is oval in shape, which may lead to arthritis around the age of 40 years. Most people with an oval hip are active and can participate in competitive sports and other activities. The oval hip may be more prone to hip injuries that could need surgery to repair, but most people with an oval hip do not need to restrict their activities. Eventually, everyone with an oval hip will need a total hip replacement[4] but most put up with very mild hip limitations until after the age of 50.

The worst residual hips are flat or saddle-shaped. These may work okay for a while during adolescence, but most become pain-

---

[4] Total hip replacement surgery replaces the ball at the top of the thigh bone with an implant.

ful before the age of 20 years. Surgical procedures such as femoral head reshaping and femoral head resection are sometimes used in an attempt to restore the round shape during the residual stage. These hold great promise, but are only performed in a few academic research centers at the time of this writing.

Stage Influences Treatment

Early in the course of Perthes, containment of the ball in the socket may help maintain its round shape. Containment is only effective until the middle part of the fragmentation stage. Numerous research studies have shown that containment needs to be performed before the outer edge of the ball has collapsed and before 20 percent of the ball has shifted outside the hip socket. Collapse does not happen to every child with Perthes, but it is a serious problem when it occurs. The goal of containment treatment is to prevent the development of a permanently flat ball, so it must be performed while the ball can be placed back into the socket. Sometimes an arthrogram (x-ray with dye) is performed under anesthesia to see if the ball can be contained in the socket or if there is hinge abduction.

Hinge Abduction

Hinge abduction means the ball is out of shape and catches on the edge of the socket when the thigh moves away from the midline. Early treatment of Perthes aims to prevent hinge abduction from occurring. When hinge abduction is present, containment rarely succeeds. After the ball has become flat and cannot go into the socket, treatment options are limited to salvage procedures. (See Chapter 5, "Remedial Procedures" on page 58.) The best way to avoid salvage procedures is to decide as early as possible whether to contain the hip because containment needs to be performed before the fragmentation stage is ending.

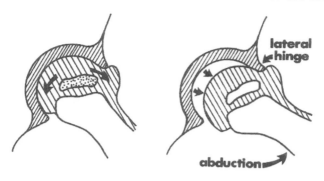

lateral
hinge

abduction

Figure 9. Hinge abduction.

Extent of Perthes: How Much of the Ball Is Affected

One of the major difficulties for doctors is to find out how much of the ball is affected in time to decide on the most effective treatment. Treatment early in the course of Perthes leads to much better results, so it is helpful to know as soon as possible how severely the hip is affected. The problem is that in the early stages of Perthes, no tests can show how much of the ball is involved, or predict how bad the Perthes will become. It's discouraging to discover that the ball has collapsed and shifted, because by then it is usually too late to restore the normal shape of this ball and socket joint.

Research is being directed towards early imaging methods to find out how much of the ball is involved, but MRI without contrast, bone scans, and other studies are not currently reliable for this purpose. In 2014, a method called Perfusion MRI was shown to accurately predict the amount of involvement during the early stages of Perthes.[5] This is an enhanced MRI technique that shows where the blood is still flowing in the ball of the

---

[5] Harry Kim, et al. "Perfusion MRI in Early Stage of Legg-Calvé-Perthes Disease to Predict Lateral Pillar Involvement: A Preliminary Study." *Journal of Bone & Joint Surgery, American,* 96(14) (2014 Jul): 1152–60.

femur (femoral head). Another approach is to wait and watch to see how bad Perthes becomes and then treat the severe cases, even though treatment is delayed by this method. However, some warning signs signal the need for early treatment even when the amount of involvement isn't known. That's because some children are at great risk for severe Perthes even when a tiny portion of the ball is involved. This chapter discusses some of the clues that help us make early decisions before it's too late.

Very young children can tolerate large amounts of involvement, but older children do not tolerate any involvement. Too often, doctors seem to observe older children and rush to treat younger children when the opposite is a more reasonable approach. (For more information, see "Age Influences Treatment and Outcome" on page 24.)

Age of the Child at Onset

Studies of untreated children from decades ago have clearly shown that children younger than five years of age at onset of pain or limp rarely develop arthritis before the age of fifty, even without treatment. More recent research shows that good results can be expected in children younger than six years whether they have surgery or are managed without surgery. In contrast, children older than nine years when their pain begins will uniformly have early, severe arthritis unless they are treated. More recent studies suggest that children older than eight years are more likely to have poor outcomes. One report showed that for 99 percent of children older than eight years, the ball collapsed to the point where surgery would be recommended.[6]

Right away, you can see that children who are nine or older, and most children eight or older, should probably be treated as soon as the diagnosis is made and before the fragmentation stage

---

[6] John A. Herring, Hui Taek Kim, and Richard Browne, "Legg-Calvé-Perthes Disease: Part II: Prospective Multicenter Study of the Effect of Treatment on Outcome," *Journal of Bone & Joint Surgery, American*, 86(10) (2004 Oct): 2121, http://jbjs.org/article.aspx?articleid=26222.

begins. Waiting for the ball to collapse or shift in the socket for the child eight or older rarely benefits a child because poor results occur without containment treatment.

A panel of Perthes experts was asked, "Should children older than eight years be treated by containment treatment as soon as the disease is diagnosed regardless of the extent of involvement?" Six agreed completely, three agreed with minor variations, and one disagreed. (For more information, see "Expert Opinions for Early Stage Treatment" on page 34.) Results are better when containment is performed as early as possible for children who are at greatest risk, especially those eight or older at time of initial diagnosis.

Most children with Perthes are age six to eight at onset, so they fall between the two age groups of younger than six and older than eight. When large studies are conducted and averages are made from the results, this middle group represents the most patients, so averaging all the age groups together creates a false sense of how to treat the child younger than six and older than eight years at onset. Unfortunately, some studies have added in the results for children under six and children eight years and older in the same analysis. Then the younger and older children are averaged into the entire group when they represent a different course of disease than the middle group.

This type of statistical error is illustrated by the following example. Suppose a flu virus causes an illness, but this type of flu never occurs before the age of six years, while half of the children between ages six and eight will get the flu, and all of the children between eight and twelve years will get the flu during the school year. Now, imagine that a school has 100 children less than six years old, 800 children between six and eight years, and 100 children between eight and twelve years. This adds up to 1,000 children. During the school year, 500 children, or half the children in the school catch that flu virus. The school could tell parents that their child has a 50:50 chance of catching this virus, or the school could tell parents of the younger children that they have nothing to worry about while all of the children older than eight should be vaccinated or else they will get sick.

Unfortunately, this is exactly the case with Perthes, but all too often the younger group gets treated like the middle group and so does the older group. It's important to separate out the middle group because their development is different from older and younger children. Not all the children in the middle group need treatment, and it may be difficult to predict who needs treatment in that group, but treatment plans are much more clear for children younger than six and older than eight years old.

The middle group is the most difficult group because this is where the extent of involvement seems to play the biggest role. Classification systems have been developed to help make treatment decisions, and several more classifications have been proposed, but none has been shown to be consistent or reliable during the early stages of Perthes when the important treatment decisions need to be made. (For information about the classifications, see "Perthes Classifications" on page 37.)

Age Influences Treatment and Outcome

When Perthes develops in a child younger than five or six years old, treatment is rarely needed and surgery does not seem to be better than non-surgical management. These younger children may continue their normal activities except for organized sports. Pain relief with medicine such as ibuprofen plus short periods of rest will help them when they have done too much. The hip stays round in 80 to 90 percent of cases, but treatment has not been shown to affect the results in this age group.

The problem for children younger than five to six years old, is that severe Perthes may damage the growth plate just below the ball of the hip. There is no known way to prevent this from happening and containment or surgery does not change the risk or result. The ball does not collapse, but the leg may become shorter on that side as the child grows. Also, the femoral neck that connects the ball to the rest of the thigh bone may not grow as long as it should. A short neck is called coxa brevis.

The growth disturbance from Perthes does not cause arthritis, but it may cause limp and shortening, and these problems are best treated at an older age. Containment does not protect the growth plate, so containment would not have helped this child who had onset before the age of five years.

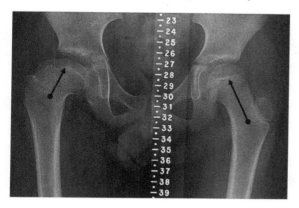

Figure 10. Coxa brevis, a short neck below the ball.

Figure 10 is an x-ray of a nine-year-old boy who developed Perthes when he was four and a half. The distance between the growth plate and the start of the shaft of the thigh bone is shorter on the side that had Perthes. The growth plate at the tip of the arrow is visible on both sides, but the affected side is irregular and thinner. The ball is large but nearly round. This shape of the ball is not likely to cause arthritis or pain until the age of 50 years or older, but this boy may need surgery to help his limp or to correct any leg length difference around age 13.

The growth disturbance from Perthes does not cause arthritis, but it may cause limp and shortening, and these problems are best treated at an older age. Containment does not protect the growth plate, so containment would not have helped this child who had onset before the age of five years.

Children eight years of age or older at the time of diagnosis should probably begin containment treatment as early as possible. Some surgeons use bone age, also called skeletal age. When this is used, the skeletal age lags behind the birth age of children.

When doctors use skeletal age, a skeletal age of more than seven years requires intervention as early as possible. Girls are more mature than boys, so the time to intervene early for girls is when they are older than seven years or they have a skeletal age older than six years.

For boys between the age of six and eight or girls between five and seven, doctors often observe the child for a period of time to see how much of the ball is involved. The child is treated for pain and limp with limitation of activities and over-the-counter pain medicines. Sometimes a period of bed rest, traction, or cast immobilization is recommended to help relieve the pain and to restore movement. However, the x-rays should be watched carefully for early changes in the outer margin of the ball. At the first signs of collapse of the outer margin of the ball or the first signs that the ball is flattening and slipping out of the socket, then containment is usually needed. See Figure 5 on page 10 to identify the break in Shenton's line that shows the ball is starting to move out of the socket.

The most common containment method is surgery to reposition the bones around the hip. Several large studies have shown that surgery is more successful than braces or physical therapy.[7, 8]

However, some doctors use one or more of the following treatments: vigorous physical therapy, braces, prolonged casting, bed rest with traction to pull on the leg, minor outpatient surgical procedures to relax tight muscles. There are reports of successful treatment by non-surgical methods and intensive physical therapy, but numerous centers in multiple countries have reported that the best results are obtained with surgical containment for the children who need treatment.

Children younger than six are a special group, as mentioned previously. These younger children have a high likelihood of

---

[7] John A. Herring, Hui Taek Kim, and Richard Browne, "Legg-Calvé-Perthes Disease: Part II: Prospective Multicenter Study of the Effect of Treatment on Outcome," *Journal of Bone & Joint Surgery, American*, 86A(10) (2004 Oct): 2121.
[8] Harry K. W. Kim, "Legg-Calvé-Perthes Disease," *Journal of the American Academy of Orthopaedic Surgeons*, 18(11) (2010): 676.

developing a round ball and treatment has not been shown to have any effect in this age group. Those who develop a slightly oval hip still have plenty of growth remaining to adjust the socket to the shape of the oval ball. This means that arthritis or limited activities from the shape of the ball are uncommon until the age of 50 years or older.

The big problem with this younger age group is that sometimes the loss of circulation damages the growth plate of the upper thigh bone. This means that some children less than six will have problems later, but early treatment has no effect on that problem. It's best to let these younger children play and be happy, because containment is not helpful, but they should be followed to see if later surgery will be needed. The good news is that the ball will stay round, unlike the older group where the ball may become flat and misshapen.

Perthes Outcome Case 1:
A Six-Year-Old Boy with Mild Perthes

This boy's only treatment was rest and the use of crutches as needed. He was allowed to walk when he felt comfortable. He was monitored with x-rays. His symptoms never got worse and went away in two and a half years. This child recovered fully. At age twelve, the ball is round and centered in the socket. He has normal activities and no arthritis is expected.

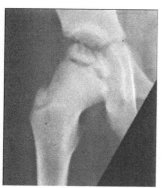

Note the moth-eaten appearance of the top of the ball of the hip.

Figure 11.   Case 1, x-ray of a six-and-a-half-year-old with hip pain and limp for two months.

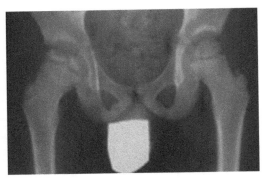

Figure 12. Case 1, this x-ray four months later shows little change.

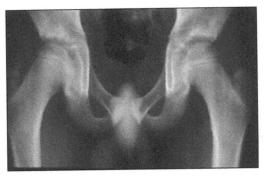

Figure 13. Case 1, at age 12, the boy's hip has fully recovered.

Perthes Outcome Case 2:
A Seven-Year-Old Boy with Severe Perthes

In this case, the entire top of the ball was involved compared to the boy in Case 1 in which only part of the ball was affected. This child's treatment was physical therapy and restriction of activities. No containment treatment was used, and the ball collapsed. The final result is a ball that is not round and will cause arthritis at a young age. This is a poor result from treatment that was limited to physical therapy and restriction of activities.

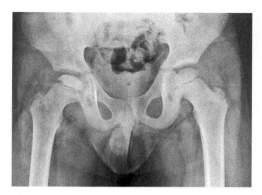

The hip on your left has Perthes. The ball is round and tall but it is whiter than the other hip and has a crack at the surface of the ball. The crack is painful like a small fracture.

Figure 14. Case 2, x-ray of a seven-and-a-half-year-old with Perthes two months after onset of pain and limp.

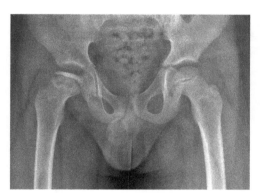

The ball has collapsed and flattened.

When a child is followed without containment treatment until the ball collapses this amount, it is very hard to return the ball to a round shape.

Figure 15. Case 2, seven months later.

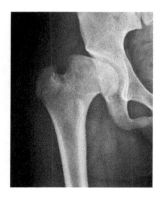

The ball is not round and it cannot rotate in the socket properly.

Figure 16.   Case 2, this x-ray was taken at the age of 17. This boy was seen because of pain and limited movement of the hip.

Perthes Outcome Case 3:
A Ten Year Old Boy Who Had a Shelf Procedure

This boy with Perthes was seen at 10 years and 4 months and was treated right away with a shelf procedure. A shelf procedure is hip surgery that adds support to the hip socket above the ball. (See "Supportive (Shelf Procedure) Pelvic Osteotomy" on page 52.) Most children in this age group will have a very poor result with arthritis as a teenager unless treatment begins before the ball starts to collapse.

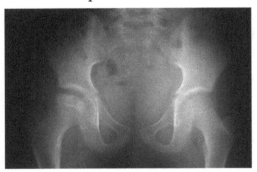

The hip on your left has Perthes. The ball on that side is whiter, shorter, and has a slightly irregular surface.

Figure 17. Case 3, initial x-ray two months after onset of pain in the right hip.

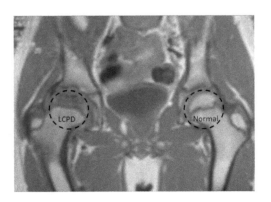

The affected ball on your left is darker than the ball on your right. This dark area on the MRI means that the ball has lost its blood supply.

Figure 18. Case 3, an MRI of both hips confirmed the diagnosis because it was an early stage Perthes and difficult to be certain from the first x-ray.

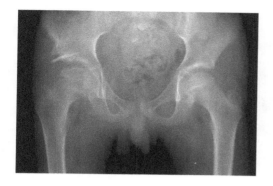

Figure 19. Case 3, x-ray of the hips after the shelf procedure was done.

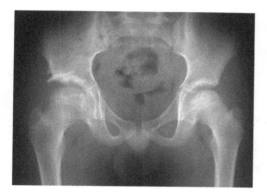

On the hip on your left, some bone is sticking out of the side of the socket. This helps support the ball during the recovery stages.

Figure 20. Case 3, x-ray at age 11 years and 4 months. The hip on your left is staying in the socket but the other hip is white and has become painful.

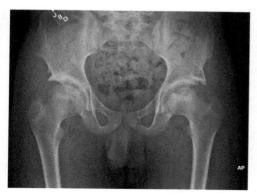

Now the opposite hip (on your right) has Perthes. Both hips become involved in about one out of six patients.

Figure 21. Case 3, x-ray at age 16 years shows that both hips are recovering nicely.

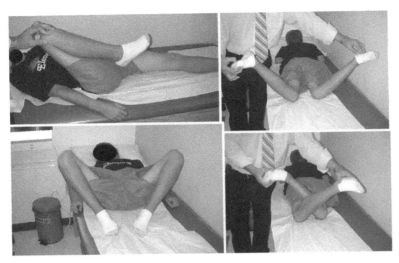

Figure 22. Case 3, these photographs show full recovery of painless movement of both hips.

Perthes Outcome Case 4:
A Six-Year-Old Boy Treated with a Varus Osteotomy

First seen at six years and four months, this boy was initially observed, and then treated with a varus osteotomy. (See "Varus Femoral Osteotomy" on page 48.) Waiting a few months to see what is going to happen is an option in the age group from the fifth birthday to the eighth birthday.

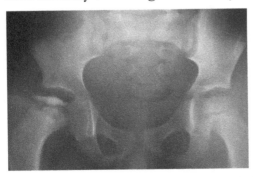

Figure 23. Case 4, the x-ray shows that the hip on your left has started to move out of the socket and the ball is collapsing.

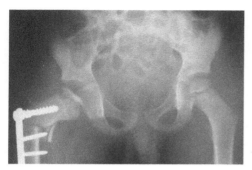

The metal pins from the surgery show as bright white on the x-ray.

Figure 24. Case 4, after surgery. This x-ray was taken after varus osteotomy surgery to put the ball back into the socket.

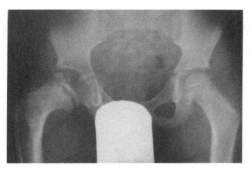

The doctor removed the metal after the osteotomy healed.

Figure 25. Case 4, one year later.

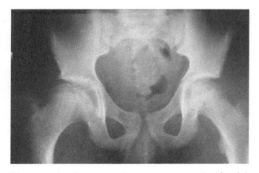

Figure 26. Case 4, at age 13 years. In the hip on your left, which had Perthes, the ball is a normal round shape with normal bone.

In Figure 26 (Case 4), the irregular area at the top of the ball is an overlapping area of the back wall of the socket, but the ball is completely smooth and round on the surface. This boy is fully active and has no pain or limp.

Expert Opinions for Early Stage Treatment

At first, it might seem like doctors' opinions vary widely about Perthes management, but the differences are not as great as it may seem to parents looking for answers for their child's problem. To find areas of agreement, ten experts, each of whom had been studying and publishing research about Perthes for more than ten years, was asked to evaluate a series of statements.[9] Each expert responded to each statement with one of four responses: agree, partially agree, partially disagree, or disagree. Here are some of the statements and the responses from the doctors:

Time Frame as a Guide to Treatment Choices

For the following statement, nine of ten experts agreed and one had partial disagreement with the terminology.

> The treatment of Perthes needs to be divided into three distinct time frames:
>
> 1.   Early in the course of the disease from onset to early fragmentation.
>
> 2.   Late in course of disease from late fragmentation to complete filling in of the femoral head (ball) with new bone.
>
> 3.   After complete healing when the final shape of the ball and hip socket are clearly established.

For the following statements, six of ten experts agreed completely, two partially agreed, and two partially disagreed. None disagreed completely. The responses are for treatment early in the course of disease. The early stage of Perthes is generally less than eight months since first limp or pain.

> Statements for Perthes in the early stages:
>
> •   The goal of treatment early in the course of disease ("a" phase) is to retain the normal shape of

---

[9] Benjamin Joseph and Charles T. Price, "Consensus Statements on the Management of Perthes Disease," *Orthopedic Clinics of North America*, 42(3) (2011 Jul): 437-440.

the femoral head (ball) by containing the ball as early as possible in patients at risk of a poor outcome.

- Containment may be achieved by nonoperative or operative means and surgical options include femoral and/or pelvic surgery.

For the following statements, nine of ten experts agreed completely and one disagreed.

Statements about containment:

- For containment to be successful, it should be achieved before the late stage of fragmentation.
- Children less than five years of age at onset of symptoms seldom need treatment regardless of extent of involvement except when the femoral head (ball) has moved out of the socket as determined by a break in Shenton's line or migration of more than 20 percent of the femoral head beyond the lateral margin of the acetabulum [hip socket].

For the following statements, five of ten experts agreed, three agreed with minor variations, and three disagreed in part.

Statements for children five years or older but less than eight years of age at time of onset of Perthes:

- Early containment [soon after diagnosis] is warranted if it can be determined that more than half the ball is abnormal.
- If early determination cannot be made, then x-rays every four months are warranted to look for early movement of the ball out of the socket.
- For those children who are being observed, containment treatment should be considered as soon as movement out of the socket is detected, provided that the disease has not progressed to the late fragmentation stage. Movement out of the socket is defined as a break in Shenton's line or more than 20% of the ball out of the socket.

- No containment in this age group is needed when the ball does not move out of the socket.

- Children eight years or older but less than twelve years of age at onset of disease should be treated by containment as soon as Perthes is diagnosed regardless of extent of necrosis. Methods other than containment should be considered when the patient has already progressed to the late fragmentation stage of disease.

For the following statement, five of ten experts agreed and five agreed with minor variations.

Statement about older children:

Children twelve years of age or older should not be treated by containment and treatment should be similar to adults with osteonecrosis [AVN].

Summary

The early stage of Perthes is generally less than eight months since first limp or pain.

Summary statements regarding treatment:

- **Less than five years old:** No treatment. Restrict from organized sports.

- **Five, six, and seven years old:**
  Begin containment treatment as early as possible when it can be determined that the extent of disease involves more than half of the ball. When the extent cannot be determined, observe for a period of time and contain the hip if there is evidence of lateral sliding of the ball from the socket (look to see if the ball is moving upward in the socket with disruption of Shenton's line, or look for more than one fifth of the ball outside the edge of the socket).

- **Eight to twelve years old:** Begin containment treatment as soon as the diagnosis has been made.

Waiting or observing is not recommended because poor outcomes will happen more than 90
percent of the time without containment, and
outcomes are best when containment begins
early for those who are at greatest risk. Surgery
usually gives better outcomes than non-surgical
treatments in this age group especially.

- **Age twelve and older:** Containment treatment
does not help these older children and adolescents. Use other methods similar to treatments
for adults.

Perthes Classifications

These classifications are mainly useful as research tools because
in most cases, it is not possible to use them to classify Perthes
during the early stages when most treatment decisions need to be
made. Reliance on classifications during early stages of Perthes
has made it hard to identify the most effective treatments early
in the course of Perthes. However, if a child is first diagnosed at
a later stage of Perthes and the femoral head already collapsed,
lateral classification is useful in predicting the future outcome of
the hip. The common classification systems are as follows:

- **Herring classification (also called Lateral Pillar classification).** This classification describes the amount of collapse
of the lateral pillar. The lateral pillar is the part of the ball
nearest the edge of the socket. Perthes is more severe when
the lateral pillar collapses.

- **Catterall classification.** This classification uses Group I
through Group IV to identify differences in the extent of
dead bone caused by Perthes that can be seen in x-rays. Less
than half of the ball is affected for Groups I and II and more
than half of the ball is affected in Groups III and IV.

- **Salter-Thompson classification.** This classification describes
two groups based on the percentage of the ball that is
involved. This depends on being able to see the crack at the
surface of the ball on early x-rays. This is sometimes helpful

during the necrosis stage, but the crack may not be visible on x-ray.

These classifications are based on the amount of ball involvement, especially the outer margin of the ball where collapse is most harmful because the ball can then slip out of the socket. The most popular of these is the Herring (also called Lateral Pillar) classification. As long as the outer margin of the ball keeps its height, then the hip cannot slip out of the socket and the ball is likely to remain round after Perthes runs its course. Remember that this classification is not helpful for the child older than eight or the child younger than five, but it may have some usefulness for the middle group between ages five and eight.

The major problem with the Catterall classification and the Lateral Pillar classification is that they are only accurate during the fragmentation stage and that's too close to the time when containment may not help.

Professor Robert Salter and George Thompson tried to classify Perthes earlier, during the necrosis stage, by looking at the length of the crack that develops under the joint surface when the child is first diagnosed. If this crack can be seen clearly, and it goes beyond the midpoint of the ball, then a lot of the ball is involved and early containment is recommended. However, the crack can't always be seen on x-ray, CT scan, or MRI. So, deciding the best method of treatment in this middle age group may be very difficult in the early stages of Perthes. Sometimes the severity of pain, limp, or limitation of movement will help make the decision. Children who have more severe pain, limp, or muscle tightness often have more severe involvement while those who maintain their movement have lesser amounts of involvement.

The Catterall classification has similar problems. Some researchers have shown that different doctors disagree on the group that each patient belongs in and there are variations of estimation of how much of the ball is affected. Also, the Catterall classification becomes more obvious in the fragmentation stage of

Perthes and is a useful research tool but may be too late to help make treatment decisions.

Containment Methods

Most experts agree that containment is only helpful during the early stages of Perthes, and they also agree about which patients need this treatment, but doctors have different opinions about the best way to manage containment treatment. The purpose of containment is to keep the ball in the socket so the socket serves as a mold to keep the ball round while the dead bone is absorbed and new bone is growing in the ball under the protection of the socket.

The methods of containment fall into two large categories:

- Non-surgical containment with casts, braces, prolonged crutch use, or vigorous physical therapy

- Surgical containment.

The choice of the containment method depends on the experience and success of the doctor along with discussions with the family regarding their preferences. Most containment methods work equally when applied correctly by doctors who understand that particular method and stick with it. Problems occur when containment begins too late or when poor containment methods are used, such as braces that are only above the knees or when containment is intermittent instead of continuous. One reason that surgery is better may be that children do not always cooperate with 12-18 months of brace treatment or vigorous physical therapy. Younger children seem to become more adjusted to non-surgical treatments, although one study shows that children treated with braces may have mild behavioral problems at an older age.[10]

---

[10] Charles T. Price, Deborah D. Day, and Joseph C. Flynn, "Behavioral Sequelae of Bracing Versus Surgery for Legg-Calvé-Perthes Disease," *Journal of Pediatric Orthopaedics*, 8(3) (1988 May): 285.

Symptomatic treatment means treating a child's symptoms such as pain. This is not containment but it can help the child feel better, especially the child younger than five to six years old who does not need containment.

3

Non-Surgical Containment

Non-surgical containment needs to be done for at least a year and often for 18 months to be successful. This treatment tends to be more successful for younger children compared to children eight years old and older. When non-surgical containment is recommended, it is difficult to start with this and change to surgery if the treatment is not working because the best time to do surgery is early in the course of disease. Surgical containment to rescue failed non-surgical management can be done, but it is usually not the best choice because it delays effective surgical treatment. It is more important to start with one method and stick with it from the beginning. Comparisons of early surgery to surgery following failed non-surgical containment treatment show much better outcomes when surgery is performed before the ball has collapsed.

Bed rest, crutches, or physical therapy can improve symptoms and movement for many children with Perthes. However, using these methods alone without containment has not improved outcomes compared to no treatment. These are often useful methods at the beginning of treatment to help improve movement but should be combined with braces, casts, or surgery for containment to provide the best outcomes.

Braces

Several medical journal articles have reported satisfactory out-comes with braces for containment. However, others have reported that some types of braces are the same as no treatment for most children. Braces are usually combined with physical therapy and non-weight bearing in a wheelchair for 12-18 months until the ball has gone through the stages of bone removal and replacement. One consistent finding is that success-ful methods used braces that extend the full length of the leg.

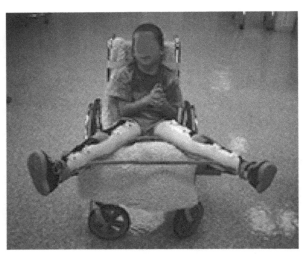

Figure 27. Child in a brace.

The most recent report suggest using an A-frame brace com-bined with bed rest, surgical release of tight muscles, and physical therapy during the period of treatment. This is an acceptable way to avoid surgical intervention but the knees must be included in the brace for best results. One study of long-term psychologi-cal effects suggested that older children treated with braces had slightly more behavioral problems after treatment when com-pared to children who had surgical treatment.

A brace is easier to manage than a cast, but it can be removed by the child so more cooperation is needed. The brace should extend from the upper thighs to the ankles or feet in order to control both hips. When only one hip is controlled, the child can twist the pelvis to defeat the purpose of the brace. The brace is usually worn full-time but some time out of the brace is allowed if the range of motion is easily maintained. Duration of wear is usually the same as a cast: for 12-18 months. Sometimes a brace is used after a cast is removed, and the same principles apply. Compared to the cast, your child can move a lot more, but it will take some time for him or her to adjust.

Casts and Bed Rest

Wearing a cast is also a successful method of non-surgical containment treatment. The advantage of casts is that the child cannot remove them. This assures that the hips will be contained all the time for the period of treatment while the ball is going through the stages of repair. In successful reports, the casts extended at least from the hips to the ankles and the legs were spread by bars that connected the two legs, because the hips are held in the socket when both legs are held wide apart.

Children who wear a cast for non-surgical containment need to have the cast changed as they grow. A visit to the doctor's office while a child is in a cast usually does not take long. After taking an x-ray to check the hips, the doctor sees if the cast needs to be changed. Discuss any questions you have during the doctor visit.

A cast saw is used to remove the cast. This is noisy and may scare some children, but it does not hurt the child. Then the doctor applies a new cast. The shape of the hole in the cast could be larger or smaller than the previous cast. Each cast is different because they are "hand-made," and the needs of the child may also change. Sometimes, cast changes are done under general anesthesia in combination with a hip arthrogram or range of movement under anesthesia. The doctor tells you when to come back for the next cast checkup.

Bisphosphonates (BPs)

All bones go through an ongoing process called remodeling in which old bone dissolves and new bone grows. Bisphosphonates (BPs), also called diphosphonates, are drugs that slow down or prevent bone from dissolving. These drugs have been used to treat conditions that involve bone loss such as osteoporosis and Paget's disease. These medication are typically taken in pill form. Use for Perthes is controversial until more research proves the benefits are greater than the risks.

4

Surgical Containment

The majority of doctors who treat Perthes prefer surgical containment when containment is needed. While it is possible to achieve satisfactory results with non-surgical methods such as braces or casts, several research studies have confirmed that surgery is more likely to provide the best outcomes. A comprehensive analysis of Perthes literature was published in 2012 and determined that children older than six years were nearly twice as likely to have a satisfactory outcome from surgical containment compared to non-surgical treatments. Children younger than six years had equivalent outcomes from surgical or non-surgical treatment but many of the younger children reviewed were less than five years old and may not have benefited from either treatment.

Several types of surgery are used to help contain the hip. Osteotomy surgery moves the bones of the thigh bone and/or the pelvis so that the hip stays in place. Shelf procedures are performed to deepen the hip socket and provide support for the hip if the ball starts to slide out of the socket. Recently, some surgeons have used external fixation to stretch the hip joint and hold it in place during the healing process. Each of these will be discussed separately, but all have about the same results when applied by experienced surgeons as soon as containment is needed.

Casts Before or After Surgery

During treatment for Perthes, your child might wear a Petrie cast (also called a Bachelor cast) or a spica cast to keep the hips in the correct position. A child can wear a cast before surgery or after surgery.

A child casted before surgery wears Petrie casts and will have gradually increasing width between the legs (abduction) to restore the hip's range of motion and push the hip into the socket. The child may wear a cast for six to eight weeks, and typically will not wear another cast after surgery.

A child who is casted after containment surgery wears a spica cast for four to six weeks. The cast helps keep the hip in place and inactive so the muscles stay relaxed. Casts aren't so much to protect the bone that is healing as they are to maintain hip joint position for a few weeks.

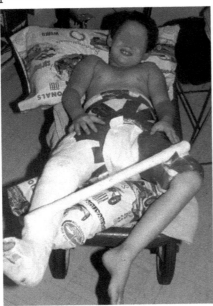

Figure 28. This boy is wearing a spica cast.

Without recovery of motion prior to surgery, the muscles are tight and in spasm. The spasms relax under general anesthesia but come back immediately after awakening. These muscle spasms may defeat the surgery unless a cast is applied until the muscle spasms settle down.

Sometimes it's possible to avoid casts after surgery by using casts, traction, bed rest or a combination of all three to get rid of muscle spasms before surgery. The doctor will advise you whether casts are needed before or after surgery, or occasionally not at all, but this is uncommon.

Traction Before Surgery

Traction is used before surgery for some children. Traction is a system of weights and pulleys used to gently stretch the muscles and tendons around the hip joint. This helps relax the muscles around the joint, so the surgery is more likely to be successful.

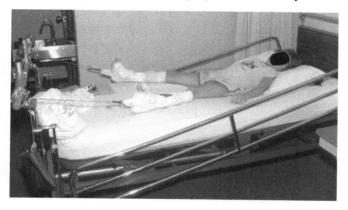

Figure 29. Child in traction.

During traction, both of the child's legs are attached with ace bandages and sticky tape to weighted ropes. The ropes go over a frame at the end of the bed where the weights hang. The weights are usually four or five pounds (about two kilos) on each side, depending on the size and age of the child. The child stays in traction 24 hours a day with short breaks. This is occasionally uncomfortable at first, but not painful. Pain medicines are almost never needed because the stretching is gradual. Both legs are included in the traction so that the pelvis can be controlled and to keep the child positioned properly.

Osteotomy Surgery

An osteotomy is surgery in which the doctor cuts bone. Osteotomies for treatment of the hip joint include pelvic osteotomy and femoral osteotomy. A pelvic osteotomy is when the doctor makes one or more cuts in bones in the pelvis, typically near or in the hip socket. A femoral osteotomy is when the doctor makes one or more cuts in the thigh bone (femur). All osteotomies around the hip require about three months to heal. Each type of surgery is described in more detail in the following sections.

Generally a cast is used for the first six weeks after the surgery and crutches are used for partial weight bearing during the second six weeks. Physical therapy is uncommon because more often children need to be slowed down than told to exercise.

If your child is having an osteotomy, ask the doctor questions to make sure that you understand the treatment. Some questions are listed below:

- Is this a pelvic osteotomy, or a femoral osteotomy, or both?
- What type of osteotomy?
- Will pins, screws, or plates be needed during this surgery? If so, how long will they be in place?
- If a donor bone will be used, where will you take the donor bone from?
- Will my child limp afterward? If so, for how long?
- Is there anything that my child is not allowed to do while recovering from the osteotomy?

Varus Femoral Osteotomy

A varus femoral osteotomy is surgery in which the doctor cuts the thigh bone (femur) and tilts the ball towards the socket so it goes deeper into the socket.

Femoral osteotomy changes the angle at which the ball (femoral head) meets the hip socket. The type used for containment of Perthes is called a varus derotational osteotomy (VDO or VDRO). Varus means inward, so in this procedure, the ball is tilted inward toward the center of the body.

This surgery improves the angle at which the upper part of the thigh bone meets the socket. During weight-bearing, the forces of the hip joint point more inward towards the center of the socket. This improves the mechanics of the hip and helps keep the ball centered in the socket while Perthes is going through the stages of healing. One advantage of this femoral osteotomy is that it is a very common procedure for many pediatric conditions, so every pediatric orthopedic surgeon is trained to do this procedure and performs it frequently for cerebral palsy, leg length discrepancy, fracture repairs, congenital hip dislocations, and other disorders of children.

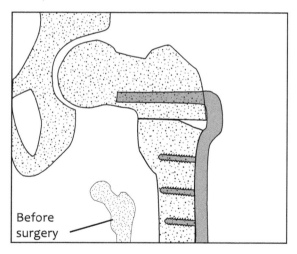

Figure 30. Varus femoral osteotomy.

Because children are still growing, the plate and screws are removed later in a separate operation, but that is not as big a procedure. (See "Removing Pins or a Plate and Screws after an Osteotomy" on page 54.)

After the femoral osteotomy, the child's operated leg is a little bit shorter, and the limp may be greater, but this is protective for the soft bone of the ball. With time the leg normally regains length because the surgery stimulates growth and children have the capacity to remodel the shape of their bones as they grow. In this context, remodel means that the bones grow into a more normal shape and alignment. One study showed that after four years, only 10 percent of children still had a mild limp or leg length discrepancy. Limp and leg length discrepancy that don't resolve can be corrected but it requires another surgery. It is more important to make sure that the ball stays round because a flattened ball is flat forever, but limp and leg length discrepancy can almost always be corrected for the 10 percent who need additional surgery.

Also, the upper part of the thigh bone can restore its shape as growth occurs. Some surgeons will drill the outer part of the bone to help the inner part grow faster to restore the shape. This is called trochanteric epiphyseodesis. Trochanteric epiphyseodesis does not interfere with the length of the leg and may help the shape recover faster.

Pelvic Osteotomy

A pelvic osteotomy is surgery in which the doctor cuts the bone in the pelvis to improve the structure of the hip socket and to improve support for the ball at the top of the thigh bone.

After a pelvic osteotomy, the child needs strong pain relief medicine for the first two weeks. Make sure that you arrange with the doctor to get the pain relief medicine ahead of time. Sometimes pins are used during the surgery. They are later removed after the hip has healed. (See "Removing Pins or a Plate and Screws after an Osteotomy" on page 54.)

The purpose of a pelvic osteotomy is to move the socket to a position that is more on top of the ball. This deepens the socket so the ball cannot escape if it begins to flatten. Pelvic osteotomies have many different names, and in some cases the same procedure has more than one name. The following sections describe the pelvic osteotomies most often performed for Perthes treatment.

Salter (Innominate) Pelvic Osteotomy

With the Salter osteotomy, the doctor tilts the socket so it holds the hip in place better. This tilting is possible because the pubic joint directly in front of the pelvis is springy in young children. This allows the surgeon to only cut the pelvis above the socket and bend it down to provide more support for the ball.

The doctor takes a graft of bone from the hip area, cuts through the bone above where the ball rests, and inserts the bone graft into the gap to hold the new position of the hip socket (acetabulum) over the ball. One or two four-inch (10 cm) pins are inserted through all the pieces of bone to hold them together. A typical scar is about three to four inches (8-10 cm) long.

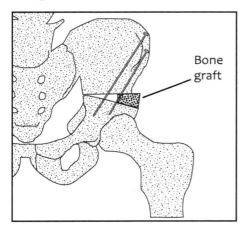

Bone graft

Figure 31. Salter Osteotomy.

Triple Pelvic Osteotomy (Steel)

The triple pelvic osteotomy combines the Salter osteotomy with two more cuts through the bones of the lower pelvis. This allows the socket to be moved more freely because the whole socket is free instead of hinging at the pubic joint. This method can be used in any age group and provides more containment than either the femoral osteotomy or the Salter osteotomy alone.

Most commonly, the triple pelvic osteotomy is used in older children or in children with more advanced stages in which the ball may already be slipping out of the socket and collapsing.

One study compared the triple pelvic osteotomy with shelf procedures. (See "Supportive (Shelf Procedure) Pelvic Osteotomy" on page 52.) The study found that the triple pelvic osteotomy was technically more difficult and had more complications, but successful cases had slightly more patients with perfect results than the patients who had shelf procedures. This problem of better results but more complications and increased technical difficulty is one reason why each doctor develops his or her own treatment preferences. It is difficult to balance the benefits against the risks, and other variables like severity, age, and progression must be included in decisions along with the doctor's own experience and knowledge.

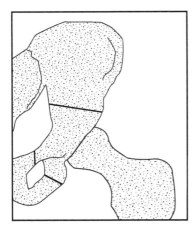 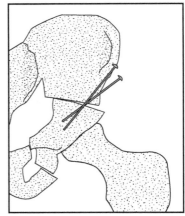

Figure 32. Triple pelvic osteotomy (Steel) before and after.

Supportive (Shelf Procedure) Pelvic Osteotomy

Shelf procedures add support to the top of the hip socket when the ball does not have enough coverage. Doctors use a number of different techniques for the shelf procedure, but they all add bone to the outside of the pelvis over the ball. This enlarges the socket and provides support for the ball without cutting the bones of the pelvis or thigh bone.

Many surgeons prefer this method for children eight years and older because it does not cut through the bone, provides good support, and does not shorten or lengthen the leg. Some pediatric orthopedic surgeons are not as familiar with shelf procedures as they are with femoral osteotomies, but this procedure has proven to be a very satisfactory treatment, especially for older children. Crutches are used for six weeks after the cast is removed. After the surgery, only partial weight can be put on the leg for three months.

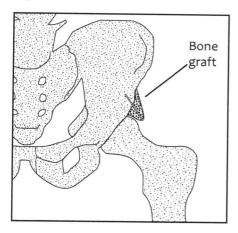

Figure 33. Shelf procedure pelvic osteotomy.

Combined Procedures

Some surgeons prefer to combine a slight femoral osteotomy with a modest amount of pelvic osteotomy. This has the advantage of keeping the anatomy closer to normal on both sides of the hip.

Like the triple pelvic osteotomy, a combined procedure is used when maximum containment is needed, especially in older children or in children who already have some ball flattening but are still in the fragmentation stage.

Most patients don't need this much support when containment begins early in the course of Perthes. The disadvantage of this approach is that the surgery is more invasive than either procedure alone. The good news is that these two procedures are not technically demanding and most pediatric orthopedic surgeons perform these procedures on a regular basis for several other conditions.

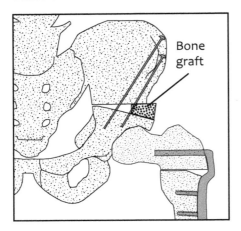

Figure 34. Salter osteotomy combined with a femoral osteotomy.

Removing Pins or a Plate and Screws after an Osteotomy

If a young child's surgery required pins or a metal plate and screws, he or she will need another surgery to remove them after the bone has healed to prevent the bone from growing over them and covering them. If bone covers the pins or plate and screws, this makes any future surgeries difficult, even a surgery in later life such as a total hip replacement at the age of 70. The length of time for the bone to heal after a child's surgery can range from six weeks after a pelvic osteotomy to four months after a femoral osteotomy. The surgery to remove metal can be planned when it's convenient for families, usually up to as much as three years after the osteotomy. After three years it is more difficult.

Removing pins or a plate and screws is normally a fairly quick surgery because it's not necessary to cut the bone again. The child usually goes home afterward without staying overnight at the hospital. Casts are not needed for removal of pins, plates or screws. Your child will be sore for a few days and probably will need pain relief. He or she might not want to move much. In some cases, the doctor limits the child's activities during recovery. For example, the child might need to stay off his or her feet for a week or two after the surgery.

Articulated Distraction (External Fixation)

Articulated distraction is also called hinged-distraction or arthro-diatasis. Surgery is used to put metal pins into the bone above and below the hip, and then the pins are connected to a metal frame outside of the child's leg. This treatment is called external fixation (sometimes abbreviated as ex-fix) because the external frame fixes the hip joint in a certain position.

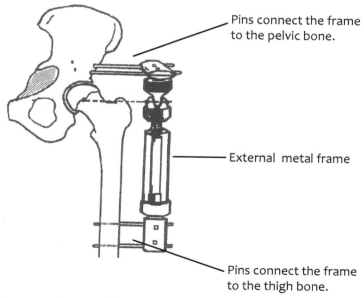

Pins connect the frame to the pelvic bone.

External metal frame

Pins connect the frame to the thigh bone.

Figure 35. External fixator.

After external fixation is applied, the child is awakened and the device can be gradually lengthened to stretch the hip joint and relieve pressure on the ball. This unloads the ball and keeps it from collapsing. It also has the potential to help the ball return to a round shape shortly after the ball has flattened. When the hip has already started to slide out of the socket, this method is sometimes used to put the hip back into the socket.

Children are allowed to use crutches two days after surgery and physical therapy is performed to help the hip move as much as possible. The separation of the joint is gradual and causes very little pain. The biggest problem is the bulkiness of the fixator and the potential for pin infections. After the joint is separated slightly, the crutches are continued while wearing the device for three to seven months with an average of four and a half months. After removal, the child stays on crutches without walking for about two more months. The total treatment time is around five to nine months.

This method may be useful for remedial surgery when the ball has collapsed and started to slip out of the joint, but is still in the fragmentation stage. A very meaningful research study was performed in Brazil where children with Perthes were assigned to have traditional containment surgery or hinged distraction. Appropriate consents and explanations were made before patients knew which type of treatment they would get. After healing and follow-up there was no difference between the two groups, but the patients treated with hinged distraction had more problems during treatment. The authors concluded, "…we do not recommend hip distraction as a primary treatment for the early stages of LCP disease." In other words, this method is not recommended during the early stages of Perthes because other methods of containment work as well and don't burden the child or family as much as having external fixation and crutches.

Core Decompression or Multiple Drilling

For this treatment, one or more holes are drilled into the ball to relieve pain from pressure and increase blood flow to help new bone grow. Core decompression is done before the ball collapses.

This treatment can be done in addition to containment treatment. Young children in the early stages of Perthes may benefit from several small holes because there is some concern that drilling through the growth plate may cause growth disturbances. For older children with more severe Perthes in the later stages, a larger hole might be needed together with removal of dead bone and the addition of some artificial bone to stimulate healing.

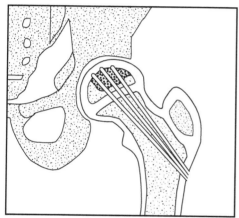

Figure 36. Core decompression.

5

Remedial Procedures

Remedial procedures are used when the ball has already slipped out of the socket and has started to heal while it is flat or misshapen. If this happens, it usually occurs during the late fragmentation stage. Under these circumstances, the orthopedic surgeon must decide if the hip can still be contained and whether the child is still young enough for the ball to grow back into a round shape. These decisions are not easily made and doctors have wide differences of opinion for management of Perthes in this later stage of disease when there is still some healing potential and the hip has collapsed partially or completely.

Remedial Procedures in the Late Fragmentation Stage

Surgical methods are generally recommended for remedial treatment of Perthes, although success has been reported with adductor tenotomy and prolonged immobilization with an A-frame brace 23 hours a day for an average of one year. Other non-surgical methods such as crutches, casts, or bed rest may relieve pain, but they will not return the ball to its round shape and long-term outcomes are poor when the ball remains misshapen.

When remedial procedures are needed, the child has an arthrogram (x-ray with dye) to find out if the hip has hinge abduction. Hinge abduction means that the ball is out of shape and catches on the edge of the socket when the thigh moves away from the midline. (See "Hinge Abduction" on page 20.) Most experts agree that hinge abduction is a very bad sign. It is best to try to contain the hip before the ball collapses to the point that hinge abduction has occurred. However, hinge abduction may occur in Perthes because of the difficulties of early decision-making.

If the child does not have hinge abduction, then containment methods described in the previous chapter may be used. In general, more complete containment is recommended in late stages as long as the ball doesn't have hinge abduction, even when the ball has collapsed. More complete containment may also be recommended in older children at the beginning of treatment because they may have poor outcomes without more vigorous treatment. Methods for more complete containment include combined procedures, triple pelvic osteotomy, or articulated distraction.

If the child's hip has hinge abduction, it is very difficult to return the hip to normal. Three methods are often used without trying to put the ball back into the socket. These are valgus femoral osteotomy (the opposite of varus femoral osteotomy that's used for containment), shelf procedure alone, or combined valgus femoral osteotomy plus shelf procedure.

Valgus Femoral Osteotomy

Valgus femoral osteotomy is the opposite of the varus femoral osteotomy that is used to contain the ball in early stages of Perthes. In the valgus femoral osteotomy, the upper end of the thigh bone is tilted away from the socket.

This moves the flat area of the ball away from the edge of the socket so it doesn't bump against the edge of the socket when the thigh is moved away from the body. After the bone is repositioned, it is held in place with a plate and screws until the bone heals. This procedure also lengthens the leg ,which is helpful for most children with hinge abduction.

Valgus femoral osteotomy is a very effective way of relieving pain and limp while helping improve motion. Long-term studies show that this method can provide many years of useful and painless hip function. This method can also help restore the ball to a more round shape when performed in late stages of Perthes.

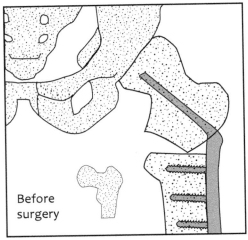

Figure 37. Valgus femoral osteotomy

Shelf Procedure Alone

The shelf procedure was described previously (see "Supportive (Shelf Procedure) Pelvic Osteotomy" on page 52). It can contain the ball in older children who do not have hinge abduction. It has also been used for patients with hinge abduction to provide more support for hips that won't go back into the socket. One report of 27 patients with hinge abduction showed that 24 patients were pain free at an average of five years after surgery. The improvement in pain and limp occurred soon after surgery for most patients along with some improvement of motion. Other scientific reports have advised against shelf procedure alone when hinge abduction is present. So, this method is still controversial but is an alternative to valgus femoral osteotomy.

Combined Valgus Femoral Osteotomy and Shelf Procedure

This combined procedure may be useful when there is hinge abduction and the edge of the socket is also worn away so that it slopes upwards. When the socket is sloped upwards, there is concern that the ball may slide out further when the valgus femoral osteotomy is performed alone. In these cases a shelf procedure may provide some extra support for the ball. However, there aren't any major reports of this combination and this choice generally depends on the experience and judgment of the surgeon.

New Methods of Containment for Hinge Abduction

Some doctors use special procedures for containment of hinge abduction in the late fragmentation stage. Other doctors recommend procedures that don't try to put the ball back in the socket because it is probably too late. Two methods that have been used to put these hips back in the socket are articulated distraction (see "Articulated Distraction (External Fixation)" on page 55) and medial capsular release. Articulated distraction has given some good results in these patients and has a lot of promise for remedial surgery in late stages of Perthes. However, long-term results have not been reported, so it's not known whether articulated distraction is better than methods that don't try to put the hip back in the socket. Medial capsular release involves opening the hip joint through the groin and cutting some muscles to allow the hip to slide back into the joint. This is followed by supportive (shelf procedure) pelvic osteotomies to keep the hip in the socket. This surgery is complex and long-term results have not been reported.

Because there aren't long term results from these methods, it is still controversial whether the hip should be put back into the socket for children who have hinge abduction. In contrast, good long-term results have been reported with valgus femoral osteotomy and this should be considered as an alternative to complex and difficult procedures until doctors learn more, or develop better methods.

Expert Opinions About Treatment in the Late Stages

Here is a summary of the questions posed to ten experts about treatment late in the course of Perthes.

For the following statement, nine of ten experts agreed completely and one agreed with minor variations.

> Containment may be considered if the ball can be contained without hinge abductions.

For the following statement, six out of ten experts agreed completely. Two agreed with minor changes, and two disagreed to some extent.

> If hinge abduction is present, containment is unlikely to improve the ball shape. A valgus femoral osteotomy is a reliable choice to improve motion and reduce pain.

For the following statement, nine of ten experts agreed completely and one disagreed in part.

> Treatment in the late fragmentation stage may be remedial or salvage depending on the deformity of the ball or presence of hinge abduction.

Remedial Procedures after Complete Healing

After complete healing, there are still some options when the ball is misshapen. The usual reason for treatment is that pain is present or the shape of the ball limits activities. This is a subject unto itself, and the variations of opinion are even greater than with remedial surgery during the fragmentation stage. There are few good options when a child or adolescent has pain and limp after Perthes has reached the reconstitution or residual stages. The remedial surgeries of valgus osteotomy or shelf procedure may be useful in some cases. However, one procedure called femoral head reshaping is being performed more frequently than in the past. Sometimes the edges of the ball are trimmed down and the socket is reshaped. This is called osteoplasty and peri-acetabular osteotomy (PAO).

Reshaping the Femoral Head

This treatment can be used for some children after Perthes has healed, but the ball (femoral head) is too large and the wrong shape to fit in the socket. In this procedure, the hip is carefully and surgically dislocated from the joint while taking great care to preserve the blood vessels to the hip. The doctor removes a section from the middle of the ball and joins the two outside halves together. This procedure has only been performed a few times and only by the most advanced surgeons in the world. Remarkable results have been reported in some cases, but long-term results are unknown.

Osteoplasty and Peri-Acetabular Osteotomy (PAO)

With this procedure, the doctor trims down the ball so it can fit into the socket better. Like the reshaping of the femoral head, this procedure is only performed by highly advanced surgeons and the long-term results are unknown. The hip is surgically dislocated so that the doctor can see the entire ball. The doctor trims down the protruding edges to make the ball rounder so that it can fit into the socket. Then the socket is realigned to support the ball. The procedure to realign the socket is called a peri-acetabular osteotomy (PAO) and is somewhat similar to the triple pelvic osteotomy. The difference is that the patient must be old enough so there are no growth plates remaining and growth has stopped. In these adolescents or young adults, the socket is released by cutting the bone directly around the socket and rotating the socket so it supports the ball better.

Total Hip Replacement (THR)

Hip joint replacement is also called total hip replacement (THR) and total hip arthroplasty (THA). This treatment can be used to treat arthritis of the hip in adults. During THR surgery, the femoral head is replaced with an implant in the shape of a ball with a stem, and a corresponding cup-shaped implant is inserted into the hip socket. There are many types of implants, and they can be made of different materials such as metal, metal and plastic, or ceramic.

Hip Resurfacing

Hip resurfacing is similar to a THR, but less bone is removed. A metal implant is placed on top of the ball, and a corresponding metal implant is placed in the hip socket. Hip resurfacing can be used to treat arthritis of the hip in adults. If the ball is not round, then hip resurfacing may not be recommended.

Adult Consequences from Perthes

The future is bright for the large majority of children who develop Perthes. The biggest long-term problems occur when the ball is flat and stays flat after Perthes has healed. Even when the ball is mushroom shaped and large, most children won't need treatment until later in life. In some children, Perthes affects the growth plate in neck of the thigh bone (femoral neck), which can cause them to need treatment after Perthes has healed. Those who need treatment as young adults may benefit from surgeries to improve their quality of life. However, there are always a few who need total hip replacement in their twenties because of severe Perthes that left the ball flat or the neck short.

Problems with the Ball of the Hip

Most children with Perthes don't have any hip problems as adults until they reach the age of 55 to 65 years. Several long-term studies have verified that children who were younger than six years at onset may limp but rarely develop arthritis before the age of 45 years. Those who developed pain as young adults generally were slightly older at the age of onset and had a flattened ball after Perthes had healed.

The good news is that the ball can reshape itself even after it's considered healed. A study that followed Perthes patients until the age of 65 years found that two-thirds of children had an irregularly shaped ball at age eight, but by the time these children grew up, only one third still had an irregularly shaped ball. So, don't despair if your child still has a slightly out of shape ball after Perthes has healed. When the ball was round at the time of skeletal maturity (or by the late teenage years), no one in the study had arthritis at age 35, but by age 65 all had some arthritis. Even patients with a slightly out of shape ball typically do well until the age of 40 years and then develop arthritis more rapidly than those with a round ball at maturity. Children older than nine years when first diagnosed with Perthes generally have earlier arthritis than children who were younger at onset. Perhaps this is because the ball in older children doesn't have as much time to spontaneously return to a round shape before growth stops completely.

After healing, most children return to full activities, including sports, whether the ball is round or not. Many doctors can tell you about their Perthes patients who went on to be All-State swimmers or soccer players, exceptional dancers, or outstanding athletes in other sports. Time will tell whether the ball reshapes itself.

For young adults with painful Perthes, treatment methods can help restore the shape, remove bumps, and repair ligaments and soft tissues around the hip so that they can resume activities. Most of the time these treatments help, but nothing is 100 percent, so some patients end up with a total hip replacement (THR) at a young age. Fortunately, those are few and far between from the doctors' perspective, but it seems quite common if you're one of the unfortunate patients who continue to have difficulties. Repairing damaged hips in adults requires special techniques that are beyond the scope of this book, and are briefly described in "Remedial Procedures after Complete Healing" on page 62.

Treatment for residual Perthes hip problems almost always involves surgery because the pain is caused by the shape of the bones, not by inflammation that occurs in some types of arthritis. Over-the-counter medicines may help relieve the pain, but cannot protect the joint from further damage. Sometimes doctors can perform a minimally invasive hip arthroscopy to repair soft tissue or remove bumps that impinge on (bump into) the edge of the socket. Other times, more serious surgery is needed.

Problems with Growth of the Neck of the Thigh Bone

The neck is the part of the thigh bone just below the ball. Some children with Perthes have a loss of blood supply to the growth plate in the neck in addition to the ball. This problem is more common in younger children, and there is no known way to prevent it. Younger children have more growth remaining, so if the neck stops growing, this results in a short neck. Even when the ball returns to a round shape in children younger than six, the growth of the neck may be damaged.

Loss of growth of the neck generally causes some difference in leg lengths as the child grows. After a few years, it is possible to calculate how much length will be lost. If the calculation shows that the difference in leg lengths will be more than ¾ inch (about 2 cm), then the doctor can perform a minor outpatient procedure to slow the growth of the long leg. This procedure is done around the age of 12 to 14 in boys or 11 to 12 in girls to allow the shorter leg to catch up so the legs will be closer in length at adulthood.

Another problem with a short neck is that the child may limp from weakness that occurs when the bone shape isn't normal. This may cause an increasing limp as a teenager. Doctors can perform surgery to transfer a muscle to increase strength and eliminate limping. If this surgery is needed, it is done around the same age as the growth equalization procedures. Waiting until that age lets the parents and doctors decide if the procedure is needed, but don't delay the surgery too long because after the adolescent growth spurt, this surgery doesn't work as well.

One more problem with a short neck is that the upper end of the thigh bone may be too close to the hip socket. This may cause the thigh bone to impinge against (bump into) the side of the pelvis when the leg moves outward (abducts). Normally, the neck allows free movement of the hip in all directions without pinching anything against the edge of the socket. When the neck is short, this can restrict movement. This problem can be corrected by surgery to lengthen the neck. This surgery is rare and it is very technical, so it's only done in a few centers on a regular basis. However, the results are generally good because the bones can be reshaped. The biggest problems occur when the ball and socket are square instead of round, (which is uncommon when the neck is short) or when the ball is large and round or mushroom shaped.

6

If Your Child Needs Surgery

Because children heal quickly and their bones are still developing, surgery can significantly improve the hip joint structure. This chapter describes how to prepare for surgery and what is involved in a typical surgery day and recovery.

Questions to Ask the Doctor

Asking the following questions might help you to better understand your child's surgery:

- What kind of surgery does my child need?
- What would be the best-case and worst-case outcomes for this surgery?
- How long is the standard surgery?
- How many times have you performed this operation?
- Can I direct-donate blood for my child's operation if you anticipate the need?
- What kind of pain relief medicine will be given to my child during surgery and afterward?
- Can my child take a favorite toy to the operating room?
- When my child wakes up after surgery, how should I expect him or her to act?
- How long do you expect my child to stay in the hospital?

If your child will wear a cast after the surgery, asking the following questions can help you prepare for it:

- How long will my child be in a cast after surgery?
- What shape and how wide will the cast be? (The doctor might not know the shape of the cast before the surgery, but if he or she does know, ask to see a picture or a drawing of it.)
- Are there any restrictions for my child afterward? Is it all right for my child to stand in the cast?
- If problems arise with my child's cast, who do I call, the hospital or your office? Can I relate my question to the office staff, and will you call me back?

Talking with Your Child

It is best to tell children that they are going to have surgery. For young children, use simple language that they can understand. Explain that the surgery is what you want to do and that you will be nearby in the hospital.

Some hospitals have programs where the child can visit to get used to the setting before the day of surgery. Children are shown the hospital gown, gas mask, and other equipment. Take some time to explain the surgery to your child or ask the doctor to explain it to her while you are present.

Preteens can understand more than a young child. Give your child opportunities to talk about any worries or fears that he or she has and to ask questions. Explain ahead of time how many days the doctor expects your child to stay at the hospital after the surgery, and about how many weeks or months that your child will wear a cast, if needed, and how long crutches or a walker will be needed. Even if the doctor has gone over this while your child is present, it can be hard to absorb everything that is said. Discuss your plans for managing school assignments and returning to school. Also explain any restrictions that the hospital has about visits from friends or the use of cell phones.

Planning Ahead

Usually a child's surgery is scheduled weeks ahead of time. In the meantime, you can do some planning in advance that will make it easier to manage when your child is recovering from the surgery.

Planning the Trip Home and Riding in the Car

If your child is young enough, you might need a booster car seat that your child can fit into while wearing the cast. This can be hard to plan for, because the doctor might not know exactly what position the child's legs will be in until surgery. Each cast must fit the child individually, with the ideal position for each hip. One child's cast can have the legs positioned much wider apart than another.

Important: Never modify a car seat or booster seat because that can affect the ability of the seat to protect your child in case of an accident. If you borrow or buy a used car seat, make sure that it has not already been in an accident. A car seat that has been in an accident is unsafe to use again.

Children who are too big for a car seat but too young or too small to sit in the front seat can use an E-Z-ON safety vest to ride safely in the back seat while lying down. The E-Z-ON vest comes in a regular upright style and in a modified style. Two types are available—one zips up the back, and the other has push buttons on the front. The zip-up type is a good choice for children who like to unbuckle themselves. To make your child comfortable, use pillows as needed under the head and under the legs.

Adolescents who are old enough and large enough to sit in the front seat will not have a cast after surgery. Recline the front passenger seat so that your child is comfortable and the seatbelt can be fastened.

For more information about car seats and the manufacturers who make them, you can contact the Automotive Safety Program, at www.preventinjury.org.

Temporary Disabled Person Parking Placards

Consider arranging for a placard that will allow you to park in handicap parking places when your child has mobility limitations. Placards can help whether you have a child in a cast, using a wheelchair, or using a walking aid like crutches or a walker. These parking spaces are located close to building entrances, and they have extra room on the sides so that you won't get pinned in by other cars parking too close for you to get your child in and out of the car.

The placard is good for up to six months. To get a temporary disabled parking placard, contact your state's department of motor vehicles (DMV). You will need to get a form for your child's doctor to sign. When you turn in the signed form at the DMV, you can get the placard. Follow the instructions from the DMV about where to put the placard in your car and when to use it. In some states, this is free. Other states charge a fee for the placard.

Making Arrangements at School

Discuss with your doctor how long you should realistically plan for your child to miss school after surgery. If you are able to schedule surgery in the summer, your child might be able to return to school at the beginning of the school year using a wheelchair or a walking aid (crutches or a walker). If the surgery is during the school year, you will need to allow enough rest and recovery time for your child.

Most public schools will send teachers to the home if children are expected to miss more than three weeks of school. The school might also be able to develop a plan in which the child attends school part time. It is best to start the paperwork before surgery. Dr. Katherine Fan, a child and adolescent psychiatrist and pediatrician has this to say about working with schools:

> Some children may benefit from a home school program. With a doctor's note, the family can request the school district to provide a more individualized and supportive learning plan in the comfort of home.

This is especially helpful if the return to school coincides with the end of the school year, which tends to be more hectic and stressful.

— Katherine Fan, MD

When your child does return to school either part time or full time, expect a lot of questions about what is wrong, especially if your child using a wheelchair, crutches, or a walker. Some schools are better able to accommodate students' needs than others. It is unlikely that your child's school has experience with Perthes treatment. It can be helpful for the doctor to write a letter explaining what your child's needs are likely to be. Many schools have aides or other staff who can assist children who have medical needs. It's also a good idea to contact your child's teacher and explain the situation. Teachers have a good understanding of how children think, and can often help lay the groundwork for a supportive classroom experience.

Taking Time Off from Work

In the United States, depending on the size of the company where you work, the Family Medical Leave Act (FMLA) might allow you to take up to twelve weeks unpaid leave per year to care for a family member. This is the same act that covers maternity leave. This can be helpful if a child needs surgery. If your child is already attending day care, he or she can continue during treatment after recovering from surgery.

Preoperative Appointment

A preoperative (pre-op) appointment is scheduled two or three weeks before your child's surgery. At this appointment, your child is checked to make sure that he or she is healthy enough for surgery. During this visit, the doctor examines the child and goes over the planned surgery with you and your child. Your child might have some tests. You might be told to stop any medications that your child is taking, and you might be given instructions about what he or she should eat in the days before the surgery.

Some pediatric departments are set up to show children around before surgery or to provide coloring books to help them understand what to expect. Hospitals provide parents with a pre-op packet of information that has instructions for when to bring the child in for surgery, where to park, and which forms need to be filled out.

You will be given instructions about how to prepare your child for surgery. For example, your child might not be able to eat prior to the surgery. You might want to discuss the following with the doctor during this visit:

- Can my child be scheduled for surgery early in the day? (This can make it easier to manage withholding food.)

- If my child will wear a cast, what kind of materials will be used (fiberglass or plaster)?

- Would it be possible for me to speak with another parent whose child has undergone similar surgery?

- What is the best way to safely drive my child home after surgery? Does the hospital have a car seat loaner program?

For more information about casts, see Chapter 7, "Caring for a Child in a Cast" on page 84.

Surgery Day

This section gives an overview of what typically happens on the day that a child has orthopedic surgery. The Hospital for Special Surgery (HSS) has an excellent video that describes this process (www.hss.edu/pediatric-orthopedic-surgery.asp). The video is specifically about HSS, so some details might be different from your experience, but it may still be useful. Before the surgery day, you should follow the instructions from the hospital to withhold food and or liquids from your child.

Generally, this is what happens:

- Your child is checked in to the hospital for surgery. Typically the hospital staff asks about your child's health history, aller-

gies, and past reaction to medications. Your child is given a
hospital gown to wear and an ID bracelet.

• The doctor examines your child to make sure that he or she is
still healthy enough for surgery.

• Next, the doctor goes over the surgery with you. Your child
will be included in this conversation if he or she is old
enough to understand what is going on.

• Anesthesia is given to your child to put him to sleep.

• You are told where you can wait during the surgery. Your
child remains asleep in the operating room (OR) throughout
the surgery.

• Your child is moved to a recovery area to wake up. You might
be able to sit with him.

• If your child will stay overnight, the hospital staff moves your
child into a room. Usually, a parent can stay overnight with
the child.

How long your child stays at the hospital depends on what
kind of surgery is performed and how he or she responds to
surgery.

What to Bring to the Hospital

For the day of surgery, and possibly an overnight stay, you may
need a number of items. Regardless of the length of stay, always
keep the most important items with you. If your child will be
staying overnight, pack a bag and leave it in the car until after the
surgery. When your child has a room, get the bag out of the car,
or ask someone to bring it to you. The following sections offer
suggestions about what to bring when you go to the hospital.

If your child will stay overnight, bring these items:

• Child's clothing. Bring socks, shoes, a shirt, pajama top, or
nightgown one size larger to go over a cast.

• Snacks such as crackers and juice boxes.

• A favorite blanket or stuffed animal, if your child has one.

- New books or toys for child. Your child might enjoy a balloon from the hospital gift shop. If you have a portable DVD player, bring it along with some favorite movies.

- If you are staying overnight too, bring comfortable clothes for yourself, too. Sweats work well for nighttime. Also bring a towel; slippers; a book, magazine, or laptop computer; and snacks. If you are breastfeeding, consider bringing a pump.

- Some parents bring a box of candy for the nurses and staff members.

- If you want to take pictures, bring your camera.

Note: If you bring valuables with you to the hospital, keep an eye on them as thefts can occur. Also follow the hospital's recommendations about valuables.

Older children often like to bring a handheld gaming console, tablet or smartphone. If your child wants to bring a cell phone, check with the hospital to find out what the policy is for cell phones. Books and magazines are also good, though it might take some time after surgery before your child feels well enough to enjoy reading.

The following items are helpful in getting through the hospital paperwork and passing the time while your child is in surgery:

- Your photo ID.

- A folder with insurance cards, referrals, and medical information.

- A cellular (mobile) phone or change for a pay phone, and a list of phone numbers of friends and family to call after the surgery.

- Snacks or change for vending machines.

- A book, magazine, or deck of cards.

Even though you know it is coming, the sight of your child going into surgery and the first time you see your child afterward can be very hard. Do what you can to mentally prepare yourself and get as much support as you can from family and friends.

Anesthesia

Before surgery, your child is given anesthesia for pain relief and to put him or her to sleep. Your child could be given either gas or an IV. He or she might also have an epidural. A pediatric anesthesiologist usually handles pain relief when a child has surgery. These doctors have special training to work with babies and children. Some hospitals allow a parent to go with the child to the operating room.

Note: In some hospitals, a sedative or calming medication is given to children before they receive anesthesia. This calms most children, but can also temporarily affect a child's mood, behavior, and coordination.

Though the idea of anesthesia for your child can be scary, keep in mind that most children who have surgery for Perthes (or other orthopedic surgery), are otherwise healthy. This means that they are in the group of patients who are considered the most fit for surgery. The American Society of Anesthesiologists (ASA) uses a physical classification system for assessing fitness for surgery from 1 to 6, with 1 being the most fit. If your child has medical concerns in addition to Perthes, the anesthesiologist takes these into consideration.

If an older child is very scared about the surgery, he or she could be given a "cocktail" such as liquid diazepam (Valium) to calm him or her down first. For a longer procedure, children might also be given some medicine to prevent nausea and vomiting during recovery.

Spinal Block or Epidural

Spinal blocks and epidural injections are types of injections into the spine to provide pain relief from the waist down. The anesthesiologist may perform a spinal block or epidural in the operating room before the child awakens, but this is uncommon because these may be more difficult and unpredictable in children than in adults. Sometimes a catheter is left in place for continuous pain relief, but this is also uncommon in children.

Postoperative (Post-Op) Recovery at the Hospital

The length of time that your child stays at the hospital depends on the type of surgery involved and the rate at which the individual child heals. Children usually stay in the hospital two to three days after an osteotomy. The doctor and hospital staff will manage pain relief and inflammation and check your child's progress to make sure that he or she is ready to go home before being discharged from the hospital. If your doctor prescribes pain relief medicine for your child to take at home, have the prescription filled before your child leaves the hospital. Take whatever supplies the nurses give you, such as moleskin and waterproof tape for a cast. Even if you can't use them right away, they will come in handy later when you are at home.

Tip: After surgery, your child might be given a device called an incentive spirometer to help clear out his chest from the anesthesia. This expands the lungs to prevent pneumonia. If your child hesitates, does not know what to do, or is afraid, ask about using a familiar toy such as a pinwheel or bubbles instead. For example, if a child can blow 10 bubbles an hour, that works as well as the incentive spirometer.

Side Effects and Complications

A side effect is a secondary effect that can be caused by medical treatment. For instance, many of the strong pain relief medicines that are needed for surgery are known to have the side effect of constipation. A complication is an extra medical problem that is connected to a medical problem that already exists. A complication can be caused by the first medical problem or it can occur during treatment. For example, arthritis is a complication associated with Perthes, and infection could be a complication of surgery.

Doctors and the hospital staff make an effort to minimize the risk of side effects and complications and to treat any problems that arise after surgery. Some common side effects during recovery are the inability to pee (urinary retention) and constipation. Potential complications specific to hip surgery are a leg-length discrepancy or numbness. Complications for surgery in general are allergic reactions, infection, bleeding, and an unplanned return to the operating room. A return to the operating room can happen if x-rays taken after surgery show that the hip is still not in the ideal position.

Swelling

Swelling is common after surgery. If your child has a cast, it might be tight for a few days until the swelling goes down. If your child is uncomfortable, the doctor might be able to make some cuts in the cast to relieve the pressure. Some casts include a window located over the child's stomach. This gives the stomach room to expand when the child eats. For children who are not casted, ice packs can help reduce swelling and alleviate pain.

Muscle Spasms

During the first few days after surgery, your child might have muscle spasms. If a child has muscle spasms, pain medicine such as acetaminophen with codeine (Tylenol with codeine) or diazepam (Valium) is given to treat the spasms. Pain medicine might also be needed, but if the spasms are controlled, this decreases pain. Moving the child's feet during the day can help minimize spasms. Some parents have seen improvement at home if a child uses a beanbag chair during the day because it supports the child's weight evenly.

Leaving the Hospital

Your child's doctor decides when your child is ready to go home. Some considerations are that the child is healing, his or her pain is well managed, and, for an older child, he or she knows how to use the walking aid that the doctor prescribed.

You might want to check the following things before you leave:

- Have you filled your child's prescription for pain relief medicine? Do you know when to give your child the next dose?

- Do you understand how your child should safely ride in the car? If you are unsure, ask about the car seat, restraint, or seat belts that will work for your child. If you have an older child or teen who is not wearing a cast, the staff can show you how to help your child into the car.

- Are you aware of any special symptoms that you should watch for at home? You might be given instructions about what symptoms to expect and in which situations you should call the doctor.

- If your child has a cast, are the edges petalled with water-resistant tape?

- Have you gathered up all of your belongings and your child's belongings?

- Do you have all paperwork that the doctor provided to you such as prescriptions, a form for a temporary disabled parking placard, a doctor's note for school?

- Have you scheduled your child's next doctor visit?

Pain Management at Home

After surgery, your doctor develops a pain management plan for your child. If your child is in pain, try to stay calm. This reduces his or her anxiety, and helps you focus on determining the source and intensity of the pain. Contact your doctor if you believe that your child's pain relief medicine needs to be adjusted.

Ask your child if he or she is in pain, where it hurts, and how much it hurts. A child's age and personality affect how he or she reacts to pain. One child might be very quiet, while another screams. Children in pain usually want to stay closer than usual to a parent or primary caregiver. Try to make yourself available. For example, settle your child where he or she can see you while you make dinner.

Pain can be treated with nonmedical techniques, such as distraction. Distraction can be as simple as allowing a child to watch more television than usual or play a handheld video game, playing music that he or she likes, or reading a story together.

The most common over-the-counter pain relief medications for children are acetaminophen (Tylenol) and ibuprofen (Advil or Motrin). Do not combine these medications unless your doctor has given you instructions to do so.

Acetaminophen provides pain relief for mild to moderate pain and fever. It does not relieve inflammation. Overdosing a child with acetaminophen can damage the liver and kidneys. Acetaminophen is included in many cough or cold medicines. Read medicine labels carefully to avoid accidentally giving your child too much acetaminophen. Make sure that you have the right size teaspoon or dropper.

Ibuprofen is a nonsteroidal anti-inflammatory drug (NSAID). It reduces inflammation, provides pain relief, and reduces fevers. Ibuprofen prevents the body from making prostaglandins (hormones that produce inflammation and pain). As a side effect, ibuprofen can cause stomach irritation. It is best to take ibuprofen on a full stomach. If your child is allergic to aspirin or has asthma, check with your doctor before giving your child ibuprofen.

Aspirin is not recommended for babies or children unless directed by a doctor. Aspirin use in children is linked to a rare but serious disease called Reye's syndrome. Naproxen (Aleve, Naprosyn, or Anaprox) is recommended only for children who are at least twelve years old.

Some prescription pain relievers for children are acetaminophen with codeine (Tylenol with codeine) and hydrocodone with acetaminophen (Vicodin, Anexsia, Lorcet, or Norco). These medications can work very well to relieve pain, but since they are opiates, they also can make the child sleepy and constipated. Make sure that you keep them out of reach of children and throw away the medication after your child is better. They can be dangerous if overused. Your pharmacist can give you instructions for safe disposal of medication. Guidelines are also available on the website for the Institute for Safe Medication Practices at www.ismp.org (search for "throw away medicine").

If your child is taking acetaminophen with codeine and is not getting enough pain relief, notify your doctor. About 10 percent of people do not metabolize codeine effectively because their bodies do not break it down into the substances that relieve pain. If this is the case for your child, the doctor can prescribe a different medicine.

If stronger pain relief is needed, such as after an osteotomy, the doctor might prescribe a medicine such as oxycodone (Oxydose) for the child. If the child is very anxious, then lorazepam (Ativan) might be prescribed at bedtime to help him or her sleep.

How much pain medicine a child needs depends on the child's weight. Make sure that you have a medication made for the size of your child. Read the label carefully. If you do not understand it, ask a pharmacist. They are trained to explain medication and can help you dose your child correctly. Once you locate the right dose, you must measure it accurately. A household teaspoon might not be accurate. Check with your pharmacist about the best device for measuring liquid medicines.

After surgery, your child's pain should decrease each day. If there is a sudden increase in pain and you do not know why, contact your doctor's office for advice.

Incisions

An incision is the place where the doctor made a cut for surgery. If your child has an incision, it will not develop a scab. This is normal. Signs of infection include redness, tenderness, swelling, and fever. If you are concerned about the incision, contact your doctor. In many cases, the incision is covered by the cast and cannot be seen. The incision usually heals within two weeks. Your child's doctor will give you instructions about what to look for concerning any potential problems with the incision while it is healing.

The appearance of the incision scar depends on the child's skin type and the kind of surgery. For hip surgery, the scar is located in the groin area and is about 2 to 3 inches (5 to 7.5 cm) long. When healed, this scar typically looks like a crease in the skin. A femoral osteotomy scar is on the outside of the thigh and is about 3-1/2 to 4 inches (8-10 cm) and will increase in length as the child grows. It can take up to a year for a scar to take on its final appearance. If plates and screws from an osteotomy need to be removed later (up to a year after the first surgery), the doctor usually reopens the original scar to avoid creating a new one.

The doctor uses one of several methods to close the incision: clips (like staples), stitches (usually dissolving), or medical glue like Dermabond. The incision might have a bandage or dressing on it. Follow the doctor's instructions about caring for the incision site. This is sometimes called wound care. Though children are routinely given antibiotics during and after surgery to prevent infection, you are given instructions about how to spot an infection if it does occur—such as pain, redness, pus, or a temperature. If you think your child has an infection, call the doctor so that it can be treated.

If clips or stitches were used to close the incision, they are removed about ten days after surgery unless dissolving stitches were used. They don't have to be removed. You might be told to keep your child's incision dry for a certain period of time. As the incision heals, a scar develops. The appearance of the scar can continue to change for up to a year after the surgery.

Nutrition and Healing

Children tend to heal well from surgery, though they might not feel like eating much for the first week or so afterward. You might have been told to stop all medicines and supplements for a couple of weeks before your child's surgery. It is important to follow the doctor's guidelines about that, but after surgery, when your child starts eating again, a multivitamin won't hurt and might be beneficial. The American Academy of Pediatrics recommendation is that all children need 400 IU of vitamin D supplementation. Vitamin D is beneficial to bones, and Vitamin C improves bone healing. Vitamin K is important for coagulation. Vitamin E increases bleeding time and supplements should probably be avoided.

Recovery

For osteotomy surgery, the doctor develops a plan for each individual child. The doctor takes into consideration the specific surgery that is done and the child's age and adjusts the plan as needed as your child heals. The recovery process after hip surgery takes an extended period of time. This can be frustrating, but it is impressive how people do manage to adapt and find the strength and stamina required.

7

Caring for a Child in a Cast

During treatment for Perthes, your child might wear a Petrie cast (also called a Bachelor cast) or a spica cast to keep the hips in the correct position. Both types of cast are described in this chapter. A child can wear a cast for one of the following reasons:

- The child wears a Petrie cast before containment surgery and might have traction to restore the hip's range of motion. The child typically does not wear another cast after surgery.
- The child has containment surgery and then wears a spica cast for four to six weeks.
- The child wears a cast for up to 18 months as a non-surgical containment treatment. As the child grows, the cast is changed.

Petrie Cast (Bachelor Cast)

This cast works like a brace. It covers the legs but not the pelvis. A bar like a broomstick connects the legs of the cast. Children can sit up in this type of cast. It's a good idea to purchase extra pillows and pillowcases if your child will have this kind of cast. Consider using a wedge pillow to prop up your child's head.

This cast works best if the legs are abducted or spread evenly at the same angle on both legs. If you put pillows under the casted legs, use same number of pillows on each leg instead of propping up one leg higher than the other. Some children have a hard time sleeping at first if they are used to sleeping on their side.

Spica Cast

A spica cast is a body cast that covers the pelvis and holds the hip joints in place. A spica cast has an outer layer that can be made of plaster or fiberglass and an inner lining that can be made of cotton or Gore-Tex (a water-resistant fabric). A plaster cast must be kept dry so that it stays hard and firm to hold the hips in place. Cotton lining should also be kept dry. Casts made of the combination of fiberglass and Gore-Tex can get wet without being damaged. Many parents like this because the child can take a bath or shower. (See "Bathing a Child in a Fiberglass and Gore-Tex Cast" on page 89.) However, some children's hands become red and irritated from touching the fiberglass. Some doctors prefer cotton lining because it can be packed more firmly and can lessen the chance of skin irritation. Cotton is softer and provides more of a cushion between the child and the cast. Ask for your doctor's preference and the reason for it.

Getting Used to the Cast

As much as possible, treat your child as you usually do. He or she will sense your attitude and react to it. Of course you should respond if your child is in pain or needs help, but do not feel as if you have to jump every time he makes a sound. Give your child a little time to settle, just as you would with any other child or new situation. Set him up to eat at the table with the rest of the family at mealtimes.

At first the idea of caring for a child in a cast may seem like running a slow-motion marathon. Everything takes longer than it ought to and facing the weeks or months of treatment ahead is daunting. As you and your child develop routines, life with the cast becomes easier to manage.

Remember that in spite of the fact that your child's hips are the center of your universe now, this will not always be the case. There is far more to your child than his hips and far more to you than being his caretaker, as important a job as that is. Take the time to appreciate the good moments with your child, and there will be good moments, though at first this could be hard to believe. Don't be afraid to ask for help or to accept help from others. Family members, friends, and other parents may be able to provide extra support while your child is in treatment.

Moving or Lifting a Child in a Cast

When you lift your child, use care. The cast adds about five pounds, but it feels like more because when you pick up your child, he or she can't move in response. It can take practice to get used to it.

Here are some suggestions:

- If your child's cast has a bar between the legs, do not use the bar to lift the cast. This can damage the cast and could possibly affect the position of your child's hips.

- Protect your back by using safe lifting techniques. Bend your knees and place one arm beneath your child's shoulders and your other arm beneath the buttocks. If two people are lifting the child, one person supports the shoulders while the other lifts the legs.

- Vary your child's position during the day. Have him or her spend time in different rooms in the house.

- When settling your child onto a flat surface, use rolled-up towels or small pillows to support the feet or legs. Make sure that your child is comfortable and the edges of the cast do not press against his or her skin. For example, when a child is on his or her stomach, place rolled-up towels beneath the front of the ankles to support them.

Taping the Edges of the Cast (Petalling)

Often the edges of the cast have waterproof tape applied. This is sometimes called petalling the cast because of the way the tape looks. Petalling makes a smoother surface against your child's skin than the cast. It also adds a barrier in case urine or stool gets onto the edges of the cast. If the tape gets soiled, it can be removed and replaced with clean tape. Over time, the tape tends to come off the chest area. Some recommended tapes are listed here:

- Nexcare waterproof tape, available at Walmart and Target stores

- Hy-Tape, which is pink and sometimes used at hospitals for wound care, or Tegaderm hospital tape

- Moleskin tape, available in drugstores with the Dr. Scholl's items (add more layers rather than trying to pull off the old tape)

To apply waterproof tape:

1. Cut 4-inch (10 cm) lengths of tape.
2. Wrap a piece of tape over the edge of the cast.
3. Add another piece right next to it, overlapping as you go. Work your way all around the opening of the cast.

Some parents line the cast opening with panty liners to protect the tape. Tape the liners in place with medical tape. You can also try Press'n Seal plastic wrap. It is made for covering unused food in the kitchen, but some inventive parents have found it sticks onto the cast and can be easily removed and thrown out when it gets dirty.

Cast Odors

To help with odors, you can try these ideas:
- Remove any old or dirty bandage material from inside the cast.

- Use a blow-dryer on a cool setting to dry out a wet lining. The CastCooler product can also help remove moisture from a plaster cast (www.castcooler.com).

- Apply an odor eliminator or perfume that the child likes to the cast (not on the child). Use it sparingly to avoid getting the cast damp or interfering with the normal airflow through the cast.

- Completely change all the tape.

When cleaning up your child, don't be afraid to put your hands inside the cast. You might be able to put a cloth down the front of the cast over the stomach and pull it out toward the bottom.

Personal Care

You will need to make some adjustments to your routine. If your child is wearing a plaster cast, it must be kept dry, which means that baths or showers are not allowed. The following sections offer some suggestions to help with your child's personal hygiene. You can use a flashlight to check inside the cast for small objects that can irritate the skin such as dry cereal or crumbs.

Toileting

Your child might be seen by an occupational therapist before going home from the hospital in a cast. The occupational therapist recommends an approach to toileting and might order a portable commode for your child.

You can try a bedpan, or help your child stand next to or over the toilet. If the cast lets the child bend at the waist, you can have him or her sit backward on the toilet seat facing the tank. For girls, a female urinal can be used instead of a bedpan. To allow a child to wear underwear, some families have bought underwear in a much larger size, and then cut the side seams and sewed Velcro or ties so that it can be fastened on top of the cast.

Bathing a Child in a Fiberglass and Gore-Tex Cast

If your child is wearing a fiberglass cast with Gore-Tex lining, he or she can take a shower or a bath, cast and all. Some doctors limit the number of baths allowed per week while a child is in a cast. Make sure that your child is secure in the shower or tub. A shower chair can allow your child to sit without slipping.

The cast dries faster after a shower than a bath. That is something to consider, depending on the weather. If it is very warm, a bath will help your child stay cool as the cast slowly dries out. In winter, a shower is a better idea. When the cast is wet, it takes about two hours to dry out on a hot day. The water that gets inside the cast turns to vapor from the warmth of the child's body. Then it passes through the Gore-Tex lining and the cast. You can dry the cast with a blow dryer set on low. This takes 45 to 60 minutes. Your child's clothes will be damp until the cast is dry.

Skin Care

Skin irritation is common when a child is wearing a cast. If the skin is irritated, clean it gently with a soft washcloth. If the child's skin becomes very irritated where the edge of the cast rubs, tape the edge of the cast, or use panty liners around the edge. If your child develops a rash, ask your pediatrician for advice about treating it. (See "Taping the Edges of the Cast (Petalling)" on page 87.)

Though most children have only minor skin irritation, it is helpful to know how to treat a sore if one develops. For a painful sore that does not have a scab, ask your pharmacist about a hydrocolloidal bandage. This is a special kind of bandage made for open sores or burns.

Hair Care

If your child is in a plaster spica cast, you can lay him or her on the kitchen counter. Then wash your child's hair over the sink. If this doesn't work, try a shampoo cap or a dry shampoo. Braids can help keep longer hair from tangling.

Clothing Tips

While your child is in a cast, try these tips to make dressing as easy—and as comfortable for your child—as possible:

- Buy clothes a size or two larger than your child would normally wear.
- Try T-shirts, pullovers, or kimono style shirts. When it is cold, sweatshirts will also work.
- For a girl, take advantage of loose dresses.
- For a child in a Petrie cast, try pants and underwear with Velcro or ties on the side. You might have to sew these or have someone sew them for you.

Eating and Nutrition

Many children eat less while they are wearing a cast. Because they are less active, they might not be as hungry as before. It is common for a child to gain very little weight while wearing a cast. Some children have trouble with constipation when wearing a cast. When a child is constipated, she has hard stools that could be painful to pass. This might be because she is moving less than usual due to the restriction of the cast. If this is the case, check with your pediatrician's office for suggestions about how to reduce the constipation.

Some common drinks and foods that can help your child to be more regular are fruits, fruit juices, vegetables, and whole grains. Other foods, such as rice, can contribute to constipation. Your pediatrician's office should have a list of foods that help relieve constipation, as well as foods to avoid. Many parenting books also include this information. Some children find it easier to have a bowel movement when they are upright or lying on their stomachs.

Muscle Tone

Your child's doctor will explain any restrictions your child might have. Some children should not stand or walk while wearing a cast. This depends on your child's individual circumstances. Your child's upper body could become very strong from moving with the cast on. At the same time, your child's abdominal muscles and lower body lose muscle tone during treatment with the cast. This is normal, and after the cast is removed your child will gradually regain muscle tone in those areas.

Adapting Your Home for a Child in a Cast

Patti Sheeter's daughter, Megan, was seven when she had hip surgery, and she wore a cast afterward. Patti offers these suggestions for parents of older children who wear spica casts after surgery:

- You will want a reclining wheelchair. Have the hospital fit your child for the wheelchair after the surgery! Our loaner chair was delivered to us while Megan was in surgery, and it turned out to be too narrow for the cast.

- Ask about Z-Flow Positioners while you are inpatient. Our hospital used them in-patient, and then we were allowed to bring them home with us. They are great! They are moldable pillows. Think Play-Doh in a Ziploc bag. They come in three or four sizes, and we used them to position Megan in bed, on the couch, etc.

- You might want to look into a wedge pillow, too. That has been great for sleeping and for belly time. We had to have a prescription for it, but we were then able to pick it up from a local home health supply store.

- Buy lots of extra pillowcases! We had six sets (two pillowcases each set) that we rotated. They [children in treatment] spend a lot of time propped in bed or on the couch with pillows, so it is nice to be able to switch them out often. Extra pillows are good, too. We used two pillows on the reclining wheelchair—one on the seat, and one on the back—to add support and make it a bit more comfortable. We also bought some new, fun bed sheets. Since Megan was going to be in her bed so much, we tried to make it a little exciting.

Furniture

Chairs can be a challenge, especially for a child in a cast. The angle of the cast varies, as does each child. What works for one child might not work for another. You might need to experiment a bit to find the best chair for your child. Some children love beanbag chairs. For a child in a Petrie (Bachelor) cast, a stool sometimes works as a low chair.

Sleeping

It can take two to three weeks for a child to adjust to sleeping in a cast after surgery. Anesthesia could throw off his or her sleeping schedule for as long as three weeks. Here are some suggestions that might help ease the adjustment period:

- **Pain relief**. Check with the doctor to confirm the best pain medicine and the dose for your child at bedtime. Some doctors recommend ibuprofen (Advil or Motrin) or acetaminophen (Tylenol) for pain, or Benadryl to make a child drowsy. Your child could be uncomfortable while his or her muscles stretch and adjust.

- **Prop up your child's legs and upper body**. Use a rolled-up blanket or cushion under the child's legs, especially if one is dangling. As his or her muscles stretch, you can reduce the height of the props until he or she doesn't need them anymore. Also try a Memory Foam pillow.

- **Change your child's position**. Your child might not be able to roll over at first. You can turn your child over to make him or her more comfortable. Make sure that he or she can breathe easily.

- **Consider other problems**. If the child is inconsolable, the problem could be something else (not the hips). Check for the same things you would otherwise look for in a fussy child: symptoms of a virus or an ear infection.

- **Some children don't sleep as well in the cast as they did before**. One family put a recliner in their daughter's room because she did not sleep well while she was in the cast. If she was inconsolable, one of the parents would lie in the recliner with her until she calmed down.

Some healthcare providers recommend changing the position of a child in a spica cast even during the night. For a healthy child with Perthes, this is not necessary. The recommendation for frequent position changes is over-emphasized for otherwise healthy children. Doctors do see pressure sores in paralyzed patients or in debilitated patients who can't tell you when they are in an uncomfortable position. In those cases, the position should be shifted every two hours to allow blood circulation to the skin. Healthy children with Perthes can wiggle enough in the cast to allow blood circulation, or they will let you know when they are uncomfortable (mothers can tell). A properly padded and positioned cast should protect the hip and allow comfort in almost any position. Simply tilting the cast every few hours is usually sufficient, and one position at night is usually fine if the child is resting comfortably. Pain at one spot can mean too much pressure there, so don't ignore pain, but it's pretty safe to ignore comfort.

While Patti Sheeter's daughter Megan was in a cast, her family decided that she should sleep downstairs.

> Megan's bedroom was upstairs, so we moved her bed to our playroom/study downstairs. She was able to watch movies and play on the computer, and we didn't have to try to haul her up and down the stairs. The portable DVD player and Nintendo DS became our best friends! A small laptop, tablet, Kindle, etc. would have been great, too (but we didn't have those things).

Megan also enjoyed playing Wii.

— Patti

School and Peers

Some people will stare when they see a child in a brace or cast. Bear in mind that they are probably trying to figure out what the child is wearing and why. It is up to you whether you want to ignore this or offer a brief explanation. Older children might get embarrassed when people stare. Talk to your child about ways to respond when this happens. Children are often happy to be friends with a child in a cast.

For children in elementary school, it might help for a parent to come into the classroom and explain what is going on. If you are able to do this, involve your child in planning and presenting this topic. This gives your child an opportunity to express himself or herself. Children often have strong preferences about certain things—even simple things like the color of a poster.

When the Cast Comes Off

For girls as well as boys, consider bringing loose long pants to wear on the car trip home. Your child will have dead skin on his or her legs. This can get all over the car seat if your child is wearing shorts or a skirt. If the child is wearing a plaster cast, the doctor uses a saw to cut apart the cast to remove it. The saw is loud and makes the cast vibrate, which tends to scare young children. Some hospitals have noise-dampening headphones that the child wears while the saw is being used. A fiberglass cast might be unwrapped instead of cut.

Once the cast is off, the child's hips are x-rayed. The doctor reviews the status of the hip with you—the structure and how he expects the hip to grow—what has improved and what should come next. The doctor will tell you when to bring in your child for the next visit.

Your child will have dry or scaly skin. Bathing helps, and a cream such as an Aquaphor product might be soothing. For the first week or more, your child could be in some pain and will be stiff. You might need to support his or her back while until the muscles adjust and get stronger. Some children start moving right away. For others it takes time for them to get used to the new freedom from the cast. Let your child be the one to decide when to move his or her legs. If the child wore a cast for a long time, the legs might stay in the same position, and only gradually will the child be able to bring them closer together.

As a general rule, for each week of wearing a cast, allow a week of recuperation. So if a child was in a cast for eight weeks, it will most likely take eight weeks for him to get back to the level of strength that he had before the cast was put on. If your child is stiff and uncomfortable, warm baths can help. This may help relax the muscles and improve flexibility. Note that some stiffness can actually be beneficial during healing because it can help keep the hip joint in a healthy alignment.

It can take months for a child to walk normally after major surgery such as an osteotomy. Your child might favor one side and might not want to be touched around the incision site. Try to be patient and let your child do as much on his own as possible. It is quicker to pick up and move a child, but allow extra time when you can for the child to move at his or her own pace. With the increased activity, your child might eat more.

As your child begins to move, the hip joints could make snapping or popping sounds because they have been in the same position for so long. This is caused by tendons moving in the hip joint. It does not mean that the top of the thighbone is coming out of the hip socket. The sounds typically come and go, and it does not hurt your child when this happens. This is common, but if you are concerned, discuss it with your doctor.

Physical Therapy

If your child goes to physical therapy, the physical therapist evaluates how your child moves and selects exercises based on your child's individual situation. The physical therapist might work with certain muscle groups such as abdominal muscles or muscles in and around the hip joints. Some other areas that might come up are posture, gait, body awareness, position sensing, and muscle sense.

8

Perthes in Daily Life

Perthes takes a long time to run its course. Whether your child has a mild case or severe case, you will probably need to make some adjustments in the way you do things. This chapter provides some suggestions about how to deal with some common mobility issues and emotional issues. You can also read personal stories about Perthes that were contributed by parents and children.

Your child might use a wheelchair and walking aids, such as crutches or a walker. Remove throw rugs and clutter at home to minimize tripping hazards. If your child needs walking aids, before your child comes home, the doctor or a healthcare worker will teach your child how to safely use the walker or crutches. Sometimes even simple things like what kind of shoes you buy can help your child feel more comfortable.

> I buy my son Nico shoes that are as light as possible. Nico's doctor suggested air bubble tennis shoes, if we could afford them. The reason is that contact between the feet and the floor affects Perthes kids the most. When I bought Nico his new shoes he said he felt like he was walking on a cloud and the boo-boo didn't hurt. For me, the shoes are a high-priority item in Nico's wardrobe, and I never skimp when it comes to his footware.
>
> —Claudia

Recovering at Home After Surgery

Plan for your child to sleep downstairs if you have stairs in your home. Some people like to use a hospital bed for the first few weeks. A hospital bed makes it easier to change position, and the trapeze bar makes it easier to get in and out of bed. Some homes do not have enough room for a hospital bed, though.

A raised toilet seat makes it much easier for an older child or teen to use the bathroom. Some hospitals provide them. The doctor might write a prescription for it at a medical supply store, which might be covered by your health insurance. Ask about this before surgery in case you need to arrange to get the toilet seat yourself. The most versatile kind of raised toilet seat can be used both by the bedside and over the toilet. Find out if the hospital will provide this, or if you need to order it. Baby wipes might work better than toilet paper when your child first comes home. Have some on hand just in case.

Your child will be allowed to take showers before he or she is allowed to take a bath. A shower bench or chair and a hand-held shower head can make bathing easier. If you have a walk-in shower, then you might be able to find a raised toilet seat that also works as a shower chair. The physical therapist or occupational therapist at the hospital can recommend other equipment and tools to aid you and your child during recovery. Tools, such as a grabber to pick up things and put on socks, make everyday tasks a little easier.

The physical therapist at the hospital will help your child learn safe ways to move while protecting the hip that had surgery. The hospital staff should also go over this with you. After you get home, your child might need help in some instances, especially the first time he or she tries to do something. Here are a few ideas to keep in mind with these firsts. Ask your child if he or she wants help or would rather try to move while you stand by just in case. If your child wants you to help move the leg on the operated side, make sure he or she is ready and then move slowly, following any movement restrictions that the doctor has given you. Moving the leg suddenly can be painful to your child.

Wheelchairs

Wheelchairs come in pediatric and adult sizes. If your child needs a wheelchair, ask the doctor to prescribe a wheelchair that fully reclines, has removable arm rests, and allows you to raise the legs up. If your child has surgery and wears a cast, this type of wheelchair makes it easier to transport a child. After the cast comes off, you can continue to use the same wheelchair.

Your child might be able to use a wheelchair to eat with the family at the dining room table. Most wheelchairs can be collapsed when not in use. Ask the doctor or healthcare professional to show you how to push your child in the wheelchair. The healthcare staff also can show you how to set the brakes and how to fold and open the wheelchair. Pushing a wheelchair is similar to pushing a stroller. Older children can move their own wheelchairs, but there might be times when they need help, especially if they are very tired due to surgery or the effects of pain medications.

When going up a ramp, push the wheelchair as you normally would. To go down a ramp, turn around so that both you and your child have your backs to the bottom of the ramp. Then carefully walk backward down the ramp as you pull the wheelchair after you.

To go up a curb, line up the front of the wheelchair so that both front wheels touch the curb at the same time. Tilt the wheelchair back a bit so the front wheels can go up the curb. Then bring the chair to a level position as you push the back wheels up onto the curb. To go down a curb, turn the wheelchair so that both you and your child have your back to the curb. Step down, and then carefully pull the wheelchair after you so that the rear wheels go down the curb first.

To load a wheelchair into the trunk of a car:

1. If the wheelchair is too heavy for you, ask for help.
2. Remove any small parts that can come off, such as cushions.

3. Fold the wheelchair (usually you pull the seat up to do this).

4. Using both hands, lift the wheelchair.

5. Slide the rear wheels in first.

6. Load any small parts that you have removed from the wheelchair.

Personalizing a Wheelchair, Crutches, or a Walker

After hip surgery, your child uses a wheelchair and a walking aid such as crutches or a walker until he or she is cleared by the doctor to walk independently. Some children like to decorate these items. Decorations can be as simple as applying colorful duct tape or stickers to crutches, or they can be elaborate.

Companies like crutcheze.com and krutchpack.com make items designed to work with crutches. Another company called Shrinkins sells decorative "skins" that can be temporarily applied to a walking aid and easily removed later. If you like the idea of decorating, but you are renting a wheelchair, you and your child could decorate it with a range of patterns from butterflies to skulls. Then you could remove the decorations before you return the equipment.

Emotional and Mental Health

Make it easy for your child to ask questions about Perthes and to share his or her feelings . When trying to make sense of an ongoing physical problem like Perthes, some children believe that they did something wrong to cause Perthes or worry about what else could go wrong. (A monster is eating my hip, what part of me will it eat next?) Remember to pay attention to brothers and sisters who do not have Perthes. They might be worried about their sibling with Perthes and they might feel left out if the child who has Perthes is the center of attention.

Lisa's Experience As a Parent

My daughter Kate was diagnosed with Perthes when she was eight years old. She was a competitive dancer working on her first solo. As Kate practiced, she had more and more pain in her right leg. We thought the pain was from overwork or a tear of her quadriceps muscle. She rested her leg for a period of time, but the pain persisted.

Kate had an MRI, which revealed the diagnosis of Perthes. Then the fear of the unknown began. First, we took her to a local pediatric orthopedic surgeon in St. Petersburg, Florida. Though the doctors were good, as parents, we didn't have a good feeling there. We traveled to Minneapolis for Christmas that year, and made an appointment with another doctor for a second opinion. This pediatric orthopedic surgeon suggested a spica cast that Kate would wear for six to eight weeks. We weren't ready to do that. We would have had to stay in Minnesota for that amount of time and Kate would have missed school. We felt anxious and afraid, but we needed to be strong for Kate, so all this time we tried not to show our emotions.

The doctor in Minnesota referred us to the doctor we chose in Orlando. As soon as we met him, we were at ease. He warned us of the long road ahead for Kate. Because she was diagnosed late and was a girl, her prognosis was worse than for most kids who suffer from Perthes. Due to the severity of her case, Kate had to be as inactive as possible. This time period was incredibly hard on her to go from competitive dancing to doing almost nothing physically.

As parents, we knew we needed to have Kate do something to keep her mind off things and keep her busy. We enrolled her in an art class. She learned to paint and draw. Her artwork was beautiful. One of the themes in this journey was that Kate's condition was "life-altering and not life-threatening." We needed to keep this in perspective not only for our sake but for hers.

Because Kate had seen so many children with conditions worse than her own, she started a business called Kate's Garden of Hope to sell her artwork and donate all profits to children's charities. It was so nice to see her sense of accomplishment when she presented her art at local art shows.

When the bone in Kate's femoral head grew back, the results were not favorable. Kate underwent surgeries in middle school and in her freshman year in high school. Sophomore year she had total hip replacement surgery the day before her sixteenth birthday. As soon as Kate had her hip replaced, the burden she had been carrying was lifted and now it feels as though it never happened. Years ago we would never have believed that could happen. Our words of encouragement to others are to stay strong for your children's sake, listen to your children and let them share their feelings. Finally, have faith in your doctors, their medical expertise and your children that they will overcome this.

Kate's Story

When I was diagnosed with Perthes, I was a competitive dancer working on my first solo. I had been dancing since the age of three and my dream was to become a professional dancer. The MRI read a clear case of Perthes. I didn't know what that meant since I was eight years old. All I knew was that I wouldn't be able to dance any longer. I was devastated, disappointed, sad, and mad all at once.

When I had to be physically inactive, my parents put me into art classes. Art kept me busy and kept my mind off dance. We formed a company "Kate's Garden of Hope" to sell my paintings and give the money to children's charities. It made me feel good to give back to kids who were less fortunate than me.

I was ten when I had my first big surgery, which was six hours long. The recovery was hard. I had to have my mom and dad help me a lot. But I bounced back and rejoined my friends at the dance studio. I felt relieved that things were going back to normal. Maybe I wouldn't have to give up dance after all.

Well, that wasn't exactly true. When I was a freshman in high school I had my second six-hour surgery. I missed a few weeks of school and felt pressure to get my work and tests done in time. A home-bound teacher came to my house to tutor me.

As if it wasn't hard enough being a freshman in a new school, I was in pain with every step I took. I tried not to limp, but it was inevitable. When I was at school I felt like everyone was watching me, wondering if I was faking my limp to get attention. One girl even asked, "Are you limping because your pants are too tight?" I was mortified! My high school campus is open air and students walk long distances to get to class. I had to ride in a golf cart with a staff person to my classes. Needless to say, I had a rough start in my high school experience.

In August before my sophomore year, I had another surgery, this time only two hours, to remove pins that were causing me some pain. I recovered faster—one week compared to three weeks for the prior surgeries. I started the school year on crutches, which was embarrassing and frustrating. One day on the way to lunch with a friend, one of my crutches got caught on a rock. I stumbled and dropped my lunch box. Feeling overwhelmed, I started to cry. I wondered, "Why is this happening to me?" I started with two crutches and worked my way down to one crutch. The crutches were hard to use—my arms were sore and I was uncomfortable.

I was in pain with every step I took. I couldn't walk, sit at my desk, lie in bed, or get into a car without a lot of pain. There was no escape, no matter what pain medicine I took (Aleve or Advil). My doctor had prescribed stronger pain medicines, but I didn't like how they made me feel, so I suffered through it. I dreaded getting up out of my chair if a teacher asked me to come and get something. I didn't want to look different. I didn't want people to think I was "playing it up." The more I tried to walk "normal," the harder it was for me. Constant pain is tiring. It drains you and you can't concentrate. It's all you think about.

That was then and this is now. It's five months after my total hip replacement surgery in March of my sophomore year. Now I'm in my junior year, and I feel like a new person. My dad says that I look different. I think that's because I'm so relieved and I can finally be myself again. I still walk with a slight limp, but I don't feel that people are watching me. I can go up and down the stairs at school and not take the elevator. My hip replacement surgery truly was a miracle.

I've learned a lot through this whole adventure. My mom calls me a "wise-old sixteen year old." I feel I value life a little more than most kids and adults because of what I've been through. I try to put things in perspective and know that what I had is nothing compared to some of the children I've seen in the hospitals. I don't judge people as fast as others. I understand what goes through people's heads when they're suffering and most kids in high school don't think that way.

I liked all my doctors. My parents and I trusted them to make the right decisions for me. One doctor, in particular, treated me like his own family and included me in on all the conversations he had with my parents. He treated me as if I were an adult. He helped me understand that everything was going to be okay, just not the exact same way as before. I feel I am as normal as any other eleventh grader now. I have hopes and aspirations to have a career in the medical field. What I've learned from all of this is that we all have our own battles; some are just bigger than others. God only gives you what you can handle.

Donna's Story

I was diagnosed with Perthes in my right hip at four and a half years old. This was about 1968. I was admitted to the hospital for three months of traction. Parents were only allowed to visit between certain hours of the day and for my mum that was a nightmare, as she had my younger sister to look after, too, and had to get her to our great-grandmother's house, then catch two buses to get to the hospital, so I only saw her a couple of times a week.

When I was released from hospital not long after my fifth birthday, I was fitted with a brace, which I wore for over a year. After that was removed, the only physiotherapy I received was being made by my parents to walk up and down the narrow hall in our house. I must have said "I can't" a lot. I was after all only six years old, and my resounding memory of that is my father constantly saying, "There is no such word as CAN'T!" No real problems from then on. I wasn't an athletic child, more happy to curl up with a good book than anything. My hip would occasionally lock up or give out under me, but otherwise I got on with growing up, getting married and having a family.

One thing I will say about a Perthes diagnosis today, is that now you can ask your doctor questions and the choices that are available are more varied, with the parents able to be with their children the entire time they are hospitalized, which I have always taken advantage of. My daughter has had prolonged periods in hospital for surgeries and I know that when she is an adult, she will remember that I was with her virtually all the time, unlike me whose memories are filled with prolonged absences and missing my parents so much, but that was the way it was then and we have a choice now.

My femoral head was mushroom-shaped, the femoral neck was shortened and widened [most likely because the growth plate was affected]. As a result, I experienced hip pain as an adult, and in my 40's I had total hip replacement (THR) surgery. At first I was afraid to have the surgery, but my hip pain was getting worse, so I decided to have the THR. After recovery, the only issue I really had was that pre-surgery my Perthes leg was almost an inch shorter than my other leg and post-surgery it's nearly half an inch longer. It proved to be the hardest part of my recovery as my body adjusted to this.

Now I forget I ever had a problem and people who meet me now don't believe that I have had a THR. At my one year post-surgery checkup my specialist told me that I could expect the prosthesis to last around 30 years! That was unexpected and very gladly received news. He also gave me some good advice— my new hip was there to be used, so get out there and use it.

Earl's Story

As a child survivor of Perthes disease, I had a pretty tough childhood, from being in a wheelchair, casts, leg braces to crutches, but marched on through life to do amazing things despite my early physical challenges... like going on national TV and winning CBS's *Survivor: Fiji* in 2007. I became the first unanimous winner in the history of the show, and dedicate my perseverance, humility, and determination to being a Perthes survivor, first and foremost.

With great support from my family and friends I've never let Perthes defeat me as an individual and wanted to set up the Perthes Kids Foundation to give back to families around the world dealing with Legg-Calvé-Perthes Disease. It is my hope that we can all connect with one another, help support each other and share our stories. Let's keep our kids inspired!

Glossary

abductor muscles The muscles that move the legs outward.

acetabulum The hip socket.

adductor muscles The muscles located across the groin that move the legs together (inward).

ALARA (as low as is reasonably achievable) When x-rays are taken, healthcare workers use this guideline to minimize the amount of radiation used.

anesthesiologist A doctor who completed an internship and residency in anesthesiology and is certified by the American Board of Anesthesiologists.

anterior approach Surgery in which the doctor approaches the joint from the front.

anteversion See femoral anteversion.

arthrogram (arthography) An x-ray with dye injected into a joint.

arthroscope A surgical tool with a probe and a light. It lets the doctor make a small cut and view the structure of the hip joint.

arthroscopy A surgical procedure sometimes used to repair tears in the labrum (the rim of soft tissue around the hip socket).

avascular necrosis (AVN) of the hip Also called osteonecrosis, aseptic necrosis, or ischemic bone necrosis. Loss of blood flow to the hip that results in bone death of the bone in the ball at the top of the femur.

Bachelor cast A cast with a bar between the legs, also called a Petrie cast or a broomstick cast.

ball and socket joint A joint that has a ball shape that fits inside a cup shape, such as the shoulder or hip.

bilateral Affecting both sides.

bisphosphates (BPs) Drugs that slow down or prevent bone from dissolving.

computed tomography (CT) A type of x-ray in which the x-ray beam moves around the body so that images can be seen from many angles.

containment The ball at the top of the thigh bone is kept inside of the hip socket.

contralateral hip The opposite hip.

core decompression A treatment in which one or more holes are drilled into the bone in the ball at the top of the thigh bone to relieve pain from pressure and increase blood flow.

coxa brevis The neck of the thigh bone that connects to the ball (femoral head) is shorter than normal in relation to the length of the thigh bone.

coxalgic gait Walking with a limp because of hip pain.

cox magna The ball at the top of the thigh bone (femoral head) is enlarged.

dislocated (luxated) hip The top of the thigh bone is outside the hip socket.

epidural Pain medicine (anesthesia) that is given through a soft tube called a catheter into the epidural space, which is near the backbone and spinal cord.

external fixator A metal frame outside the child's leg that connects to metal pins the surgeon puts in the bone above and below the hip.

femur The thigh bone.

femoral head The ball at the top of the femur (thigh bone).

femoral osteotomy Surgery involving cutting the femur (thigh bone), usually combined with repositioning it within the hip socket.

fragmentation stage The stage in Perthes in which the dead bone begins to dissolve as part of the healing process.

hinge abduction The ball is out of shape and catches on the edge of the socket when the thigh moves away from the midline of the body.

hip resurfacing This is a surgical alternative to total hip replacement (THR) surgery for some adults with hip problems. The femoral head and the hip socket are resurfaced, and metal implants are inserted.

ischemic bone necrosis See avascular necrosis of the hip.

incentive spirometer A device used to encourage a patient to breathe deeply after surgery.

incision The cut a doctor makes in order to do surgery.

labrum The rim of soft tissue that surrounds the hip joint.

leg length discrepancy One leg is longer than the other.

Legg-Calvè-Perthes disease A condition in which the bone in the ball in a child's hip joint loses its circulation and becomes brittle.

ligaments Bands of tough tissue that connect bones together.

low muscle tone Poor muscle tone, less strength than usual.

MRI (magnetic resonance imaging) MRI uses a strong magnetic field and radio waves to create images of tissues.

medial approach Surgery in which the doctor approaches the joint from the side.

medial circumflex femoral artery (MFA) The artery that provides blood flow to the hip.

necrosis Death (of the bone).

nonsteriodal anti-inflammatory drug (NSAID) These drugs offer pain relief and reduce inflammation. Some common examples are ibuprofen and aspirin.

onset stage The first stage of Perthes in which blood flow to the hip joint stops. This stage is not visible in x-rays.

orthopedist A doctor who treats problems with muscles and bones. Also see pediatric orthopedic surgeon.

orthotist An orthotist makes and fits orthopedic braces prescribed by doctors.

ossification The process of cartilage hardening into bone. This is a normal development.

osteonecrosis See avascular necrosis of the hip.

osteotomy Surgery that involves cutting bone. Also see pelvic osteotomy and femoral osteotomy.

osteoarthritis A joint disease in which the cartilage wears away or breaks down, causing pain and inflammation.

patient-controlled anesthesia (PCA) Pain medication in a pump that is controlled by a patient, who pushes a button as needed to get more pain medicine.

pediatric orthopedic surgeon A doctor who treats problems with muscles and bones in children.

pediatrician A doctor who specializes in treating children.

pelvic osteotomy Cutting and reshaping the pelvis (bone) so that it holds the femoral head in the hip socket.

petalling Applying tape around the opening of a cast.

Petrie cast Also called a Bachelor cast or broomstick cast. A cast with a bar between the legs.

physical therapist A physical therapist is trained to work with people of all ages to prevent the onset, or reduce the progression, of conditions resulting from disease, injury, or other causes.

posterior approach Surgery in which the doctor approaches the joint from the back.

radiologist   A medical doctor who is certified as a specialist in reading x-rays, MRIs, and CT scans.

range of motion The amount of movement possible for a joint.

reconstitution stage The stage of Perthes when all the white, dead bone has dissolved. At this stage, the shape of the ball is permanent.

reduction Putting a bone back into its proper position, such as putting the femoral head back inside the hip socket.

remodeling An ongoing normal process in which new bone gradually grows, and old bone tissue is absorbed.

residual stage The final stage of Perthes when all the cartilage has been replaced by bone and the entire bone surface of the ball has been restored.

risk factors Reasons why a person is more likely to have a medical condition.

shelf procedure A type of pelvic osteotomy surgery in which bone is added at the top of the hip socket to add support to the joint.

spica cast A body cast that is used to hold a child's hips in place after some kinds of orthopedic surgery.

synovial fluid The fluid within a joint that lubricates it.

synovial lining Also called synovium, the lining of a joint such as the hip joint.

tendons The connective tissues that attach muscles to bones.

total hip replacement (THR) Surgery in which the top of the thigh bone (femoral head) and the corresponding part of the hip socket are replaced with an implant.

trochanteric epiphyseodesis Surgery in which the doctor drills holes in the outer part of the upper thigh bone to help the bone in the inner thigh bone grow to restore its shape.

traction Weights and pulleys used to stretch muscles.

valgus Outward, away from the center of the body.

varus Inward toward the center of the body.

x-ray A form of electromagnetic radiation. In a healthcare setting, a machine sends x-rays through the body. A computer or special film records the images that are created.

Bibliography

Books

Crock, H.V. *An Atlas of Vascular Anatomy of the Skeleton and Spinal Cord."* London: Martin Dunitz, 1996.

Paley, Dror. *Principles of Deformity Correction.* New York: Springer, 2002.

Trueta, Josep. *Studies of the Development and Decay of the Human Frame.* Philadelphia: W. B. Saunders,1968.

Medical Journal Articles

Aksoy, M.C., O. Caglar, M. Yazici, and A.M. Alpaslan. "Comparison between Braced and Non-Braced Legg-Calvé-Perthes-Disease Patients: A Radiological Outcome Study." *Journal of Pediatric Orthopaedics, British* 13, no. 3 (May 2004): 153–7.

Bankes, M.J. K., A. Catterall, and A. Hashemi-Nejad. "Valgus Extension Osteotomy for 'Hinge Abduction' in Perthes' Disease: Results at Maturity and Factors Influencing the Radiological Outcome." *Journal of Bone & Joint Surgery, British* 82, no. 4 (May 2000): 548–54.

Bowen, J.R., F.C. Schreiber, B.K. Foster, and B.K. Wein. "Premature Femoral Neck Physeal Closure in Perthes' Disease." *Clinical Orthopaedics and Related Research* 171 (November-December 1982): 24–29.

Brotherton, B.J. and B. McKibbin. "Perthes' Disease Treated by Prolonged Recumbency and Femoral Head Containment: a Long-Term Appraisal." *Journal of Bone & Joint Surgery, British* 59, no. 1 (February 1977): 8–14.

Canavese, F. and A. Dimeglio. "Perthes' Disease: Prognosis in Children Under Six Years of Age." *Journal of Bone & Joint Surgery, British* 90, no. 7 (July 2008): 940–5.

Catterall, A., "The Natural History of Perthes' Disease." *Journal of Bone & Joint Surgery, British* 53B, no. 1 (February 1971): 37–53.

Daly, K., C. Bruce, and A. Catterall. "Lateral Shelf Acetabuloplasty in Perthes' Disease: A Review of the End of Growth." *Journal of Bone & Joint Surgery, British* 81B, no. 3 (May 1999) 380–4.

de Gheldere, A. and D.M. Eastwood. "Valgus Osteotomy for Hinge Abduction." *Orthopedic Clinics of North America* 42, no. 3 (July 2011): 349–54.

Dimeglio, A. and F. Canavese. "Imaging in Legg-Calvé-Perthes Disease." *Orthopedic Clinics of North America* 42 no. 3 (July 2011): 297–302.

Frantzen, M.J., S. Robben. A.A. Postma, J. Zoetelief, J.E. Wildberger, and G.J. Kemerink. "Gonad Shielding in Paediatric Pelvic Radiography: Disadvantages Prevail Over Benefit." *Insights Imaging* 3 no. 1 (February 2012): 23–32.

Freeman, R. T., A.M. Wainwright, T.N. Theologis, and M.K. Benson. "The Outcome of Patients with Hinge Abduction in Severe Perthes Disease Treated by Shelf Acetabuloplasty." *Journal of Pediatric Orthopaedics* 28 no. 6 (September 2008): 619–25.

Green, N.E., R.D. Beauchamp, and P.P. Griffin. "Epiphyseal Extrusion as a Prognostic Index in Legg-Calvé-Perthes

Disease." *Journal of Bone & Joint Surgery, American* 63A no. 6 (July 1981): 900–5.

Herrera-Soto, J.A. and C.T. Price. "Core Decompression and Labral Support for the Treatment of Juvenile Osteonecrosis." *Journal of Pediatric Orthopaedics* 31, Suppl 2 (September 2011): S212-6.

Herrera-Soto, J.A. and C.T. Price. "Core Decompression for Juvenile Osteonecrosis." *Orthopedic Clinics of North America* 42, no. 3 (July 2011): 429–36.

Herring, J., H.T. Kim, and R. Browne. "Legg-Calvé-Perthes Disease: Part I: Classification of Radiographs with Use of Modified Lateral Pillar and Stulberg Classifications." *Journal of Bone & Joint Surgery, American* 86A, no. 10 (October 2004): 2103–20.

Herring, J., H.T. Kim, and R. Browne. "Legg-Calvé-Perthes Disease: Part II: Prospective Multicenter Study of the Effect of Treatment on Outcome." *Journal of Bone & Joint Surgery, American*, 86A, no. 10 (October 2004): 2121–34.

Hosney, G., "Articulated Distraction." *Orthopedic Clinics of North America* 42, no. 3 (July 2011): 361–4.

Huang, M.J. and S.C. Huang. "Surgical Treatment of Severe Perthes Disease: Comparison of Triple Osteotomy and Shelf Augmentation." *Journal of the Formosan Medical Association* 98, no. 3 (March 1999): 183–9.

Ippolito, E., C. Tudisco, and P. Farsetti. "The Long-term Prognosis of Unilateral Perthes' Disease." *Journal of Bone & Joint Surgery, British* 69B, no. 2 (March 1987): 243–50.

Joseph, B. and C.T. Price. "Consensus Statements on the Management of Perthes Disease." *Orthopedic Clinics of North America* 42, no. 3 (July 2011): 437–40.

Joseph, B. and C.T. Price. "Principles of Containment Treatment Aimed at Preventing Femoral Head Deformation in Perthes

Disease." *Orthopedic Clinics of North America* 42, no. 3 (July 2011): 317–27.

Kim, H.K.W. "Legg-Calvé-Perthes Disease." *Journal of the American Academy of Orthopaedic Surgeons* 18, no. 11 (November 2010): 676–86.

Kim, H.K.W., K.D. Wiesman, V. Kulkarni, J. Burgess, E. Chen, C. Brabham, H. Ikram, et al. "Perfusion MRI in Early Stage of Legg-Calvé-Perthes Disease to Predict Lateral Pillar Involvement: A Preliminary Study." *Journal of Bone & Joint Surgery, American* 96, no. 14 (July 2014): 1152–60.

Kim, H.T., J.K. Gu, S.H. Bae, J.H. Jang, and J.S. Lee. "Does Valgus Femoral Osteotomy Improve Femoral Head Roundness in Severe Legg-Calvé-Perthes Disease?" *Clinical Orthopaedics and Related Research* 471, no. 3 (March 2013): 1021–7.

Lloyd-Roberts, G.C., A. Catterall, and P.B. Salamon. "A Controlled Study of the Indications for and the Results of Femoral Osteotomy in Perthes' Disease." *Journal of Bone & Joint Surgery, British* 58B, no. 1 (February 1976): 31–6.

Martinez, A.G., S.L. Weinstein, and F.R. Dietz. "The Weight-Bearing Abduction Brace for the Treatment of Legg-Perthes Disease." *Journal of Bone & Joint Surgery, American* 74A, no. 1 (January 1992): 12–21.

Meehan, P.L., D. Angel, and J.M. Nelson. "The Scottish Rite Abduction Orthosis in the Treatment of Legg-Perthes Disease: A Radiographic Analysis." *Journal of Bone & Joint Surgery, American* 74A, no. 1 (January 1992): 2–12.

Mose, K. "Methods of Measuring in Legg-Calvé-Perthes Disease with Special Regard to the Prognosis." *Clinical Orthopaedics and Related Research* 150 (July-August 1980):103–9.

Nguyen, N. A., G. Klein, G. Dogbey, J.B. McCourt, and C.T. Mehlman. "Operative Versus Nonoperative Treatments for Legg-Calvé-Perthes Disease: A Meta-analysis." *Journal of*

Pediatric Orthopaedics 32, no. 7 (October-November 2012): 697–705.

Novais, E.N., J. Clohisy, K. Siebenrock, and D. Podeszwa. "Treatment of the Symptomatic Healed Perthes Hip." *Orthopedic Clinics of North America*, 42, no. 3 (July 2011): 401–7.

Paley, D. "The Treatment of Femoral Head Deformity and Coxa Magna by the Ganz Femoral Head Reduction Osteotomy." *Orthopedic Clinics of North America* 42, no. 3 (July 2011): 389–99.

Papapoulos, S.E., "Bisphosphonates: How Do They Work?" *Best Practice & Research: Clinical Endocrinology & Metabolism* 22, no. 5 (October 2008): 831–47.

Petrie, J.G. and I. Bitenc. "The Abduction Weight-Bearing Treatment in Legg-Perthes Disease." *Journal of Bone & Joint Surgery, British* 53B, no. 1 (February 1971): 54–62.

Price, C.T., D.D. Day, and J.C. Flynn. "Behavioral Sequelae of Bracing Versus Surgery for Legg-Calvé-Perthes Disease." *Journal of Pediatric Orthopaedics* 8, no. 3 (May-June 1988): 285–7.

Price, C.T., G.H. Thompson, and T.G. Wenger. "Containment Methods for Treatment of Legg-Calvé-Perthes Disease." *Orthopedic Clinics of North America* 42, no. 3 (July 2011): 329–40.

Reinker, K. A. "Shelf and/or Reduction and Containment Surgery." *Orthopedic Clinics of North America* 42, no. 3 (July 2011): p. 355–9.

Rich, M. M. and P.L. Schoenecker. "Management of Legg-Calvé-Perthes Disease Using an A-frame Orthosis and Hip Range of Motion: A 25-Year Experience." *Journal of Pediatric Orthopaedics* 33, no. 2 (March 2013): 112–9.

Salter, R.B. "The Present Status of Surgical Treatment for Legg-Perthes Disease." *Journal of Bone & Joint Surgery, American* 66A, no. 6 (July 1984): 961–6.

Salter, R. B. and G.H. Thompson. "Legg-Calvé-Perthes Disease: The Prognostic Significance of the Subchondral Fracture and a Two-Group Classification of the Femoral Head Involvement." *Journal of Bone & Joint Surgery, American* 66A, no. 4 (April 1984): 479–89.

Salter, R.B. "Legg-Calvé-Perthes Disease: The Scientific Basis for the Methods of Treatment and Their Indications." *Clinical Orthopaedics and Related Research* 150 (1980): 8–11.

Stulberg, S. D., D.R. Cooperman, and R. Wallensten. "The Natural History of Legg-Calvé-Perthes Disease." *Journal of Bone & Joint Surgery, American* 63A, no. 7 (September 1981): 1095–1108.

Sugimoto, Y., H. Akazawa, S. Mitani, M. Tanaka, T. Nakagomi, K. Asaumi, and T. Ozaki. "Lateral and Posterior Pillar Grade Changes During the Treatment of Perthes Disease in Older Patients Using Skin Traction and Range of Motion Exercises." *Archives of Orthopaedic and Trauma Surgery* 126, no. 2 (March 2006): 101–4.

Terjesen, T., O. Wiig, and S. Svenningsen. "The Natural History of Perthes' Disease." *Acta Orthopaedica* 81, no. 6 (December 2010): 708–14.

Trias, A. "Femoral Osteotomy in Perthes Disease." *Clinical Orthopaedics and Related Research* 137 (November-December 1978): 195–207.

Volpon, J.B. "Comparison between Innominate Osteotomy and Arthrodistraction as a Primary Treatment for Legg-Calvé-Perthes Disease: A Prospective Controlled Trial." *International Orthopaedics* 36, no. 9 (September 2012): 1899–1905.

Wenger, D.R. and H.S. Hosalker. "Principles of Treating the Sequelae of Perthes Disease." *Orthopedic Clinics of North America* 42, no. 3 (July 2011): 365–72.

Yoo, W.J., I.H. Choi, T.J. Cho, C.Y. Chung, Y.W. Shin, and S.J. Shin. "Shelf Acetabuloplasty for Children with Perthes Disease and Reducible Subluxation of the Hip : Prognostic Factors Related to Hip Remodelling." *Journal of Bone & Joint Surgery, British* 91B, no. 10 (October 2009): 1383–7.

Young, M.L., D.G. Little, and H.K. Kim. "Evidence for Using Bisphosphonates to Treat Legg-Calvé-Perthes Disease." *Clinical Orthopaedics and Related Research* 470, no. 9 (September 2012): 2462–75.

Resources

This chapter provides addtional resources pertaining to Perthes and children's health.

Perthes Organizations and Groups

Here are some resources that you might find helpful. Though every effort has been made to select online content that is likely to remain available, the information on websites and their location can change. If you have trouble locating a resource, try a search. Searching is also a good way to discover new information that could have been put online after thsi list was created.

The following nonprofit organizations offer information about Perthes and online support:

International Perthes Study Group
http://community.tsrhc.org/PerthesDisease

Perthes Kids Foundation
1431 Ocean Ave. Ste. 909
Santa Monica, CA 90401
www.pertheskidsfoundation.org/

STEPS Charity Worldwide (United Kingdom)
Wright House/Crouchley La,
Lymm WA13 0AS
England
Help Line: 01925 750271
http://www.steps-charity.org.uk/

There are several active online Perthes support groups on Facebook. The easiest way to find them is to search from Facebook.

Online Video Resources

Hospital for Special Surgery. "Video Guide to Pediatric Orthopedic Surgery" www.hss.edu/pediatric-orthopedic-surgery.asp#. VDGuwxZ0YUo (accessed October 5, 2014).

Radiology Info. "Your Radiologist Explains MR Arthrography of the Hip." www.radiologyinfo.org/en/photocat/gallery3. cfm?image=kaye_Hip_MR.jpg&pg=arthrog (accessed December 29, 2014).

Health and Medical Organizations

American Board of Pediatrics
111 Silver Cedar Court, Chapel Hill, NC 27514
(919) 929-0461, E-mail: abpeds@abpeds.org

Automotive Safety Program, Special Needs Transportation
575 West Drive Room 004, Indianapolis, IN 46202
(317)274-2977, (800)543-6227 toll-free, www.preventinjury.org

Centers for Medicare & Medicaid Services (CMS)

Also administers **State Children's Health Insurance (SCHIP), Easter Seals**
230 West Monroe Street, Suite 1800, Chicago, IL 60606
(312) 726-6200, (800) 221-6827 toll-free
www.easterseals.com

Healthfinder, National Health Information Center
U.S. Department of Health and Human Services,
www.healthfinder.gov

In Car Safety Centre, Unit 5 (United Kingdom)
The Auto Centre, Stacey Bushes, Milton
Keynes, MK12 6HS, England
Telephone: 01908 220909

National Institutes of Health
9000 Rockville Pike,
Bethesda, MD 20892
(301) 496-4000, TTY 301-402-9612
www.nih.gov; For publications: http://catalog.niams.nih.gov

Pediatric Orthopaedic Society of North America (POSNA)
9400 West Higgins Road, Suite 500, Rosemont, IL 60018-4976
(847) 698-1692
www.posna.org

PubMed
(a free digital archive service of the National Library of Medicine) www.pubmed.gov

Safe Kids Worldwide (car seats and restraints)
1301 Pennsylvania Avenue, N.W., Suite 1000
Washington, DC 20004-1707
(202) 662-0600, www.safekids.org

Shriners Hospitals for Children
P.O. Box 31356
Tampa, FL 33631
(800) 237-5505
www.shrinershospitalforchildren.org

Special Products

Cast Cooler helps to remove moisture from plaster casts.
www.castcooler.com/

Shrinkins offers removable decorations for casts, crutches, or wheelchairs. www.shrinkins.com.

Children's Books

Hopkins Children's Hospital, A Child's Guide to Surgery Coloring Book. At the website www.hopkinschildrens.org, search for coloring book.

Roy, Ron, A to Z Mysteries, *The X'ed-Out X-Ray*. This is a fun mystery for children from kindergarten to third grade. Can an x-ray be a clue?

Health and Medical Articles and Fact Sheets

This section lists articles relevant to Perthes that are written for patients' families.

American Society of Anesthesiologists, "Children and Anesthesia" www.asahq.org/sitecore/content/WhenSecondsCount/Patients-Home/Preparing-for-Surgery/Children-and-Anesthesia.aspx.

Agency for Healthcare Research and Quality (AHRQ), US Department of Health and Human Services, "20 Tips to Help Prevent Medical Errors in Children, Patient Fact Sheet," AHRQ Publication No. 02-P034, Sep 2002. Agency for Healthcare Research and Quality, Rockville, MD, www.ahrq.gov.

Children's Hospital of Philadelphia (CHOP) has a website for children that includes animated characters. www.chop.edu/kidshealthgalaxy/index.html

Cincinnati Children's Hospital, "Petrie Cast Care." From this website, search for "petrie cast care," www.cincinnatichildrens.org.

Heisler, Jennifer RN, About.com Guide, "How to Prepare Your Child for Surgery," accessed July 7, 2012. http://surgery.about.com/od/pediatricsurgery/ss/PreparingPeds.htm.

Hospital for Special Surgery (HSS) has extensive patient information on their website. Some examples are: "Family Guide to Pediatric Orthopedic Surgery" and "Treatment Options for Hip Pain." www.hss.edu.

Johns Hopkins Children's Center, at www.hopkinschildrens.org, click the Just for Kids tab for child-friendly topics such as My Doctor Visit and My Hospital Stay.

Kid's Health from Nemours. This website has sections for parents, teens, and children in English and Spanish. Click tabs or search for the topic that interests you. www.kidshealth.org.

MedlinePlus, Medical Encyclopedia, Dictionary, and health topics in many languages, www.nlm.nih.gov.

Phoenix Children's Hospital, Emily Center, "Spica Cast Care." From this website, search for "spica cast care," www.phoenixchildrens.org.

Index

Page numbers in italics refer to illustrations.

CPSIA information can be obtained
at www.ICGtesting.com
Printed in the USA
BVHW021313161020
591219BV00015B/199

9 781942 480006